# Walking Seattle

**John Owen**

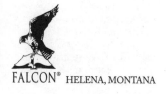

Endorsed by the American Volkssport Association

FALCON® HELENA, MONTANA

# A FALCON GUIDE ®

Falcon® Publishing is continually expanding its list of recreational guide-books. All books include detailed descriptions, accurate maps, and all the information necessary for enjoyable trips. You can order extra copies of this book and get information and prices for other Falcon® books by writing Falcon, P.O. Box 1718, Helena, MT 59624 or calling toll-free 1-800-582-2665. Also, please ask for a free copy of our current catalog. Visit our website at www.FalconOutdoors.com or contact us by e-mail at falcon@falcon.com.

Project Editor: Gayle Shirley
Production Editor: Larissa Berry
Cartographer: Tony Moore
Page Compositor: SRC Graphics
Book design by Falcon Publishing, Inc

All black-and-white photos by the author unless otherwise noted.

Cataloging-in-Publication Data is on file at the Library of Congress.

## CAUTION

Outdoor recreational activities are by their very nature potentially haz-ardous. All participants in such activities must assume responsibility for their own actions and safety. The information contained in this guidebook cannot replace sound judgment and good decision-making skills, which help reduce exposure, nor does the scope of this book allow for the disclosure of all the potential hazards and risks involved in such activities.

Learn as much as possible about the outdoor recreational activities in which you participate, prepare for the unexpected, and be cautious. The reward will be a safer and more enjoyable experience.

To Alice, my walking buddy

# Contents

### the walks

### of interest

# Foreword

For almost twenty years, Falcon has guided millions of people to America's wild outside, showing them where to paddle, hike, bike, bird, fish, climb, and drive. With this walking series, we at Falcon ask you to try something just as adventurous. We invite you to experience this country from its sidewalks, not its back roads, and to stroll through some of America's most interesting cities.

In their haste to get where they are going, travelers often bypass this country's cities, and in the process, they miss the historic and scenic treasures hidden among the bricks. Many people seek spectacular scenery and beautiful settings on top of the mountains, along the rivers, and in the woods. While nothing can replace the serenity and inspiration of America's natural wonders, we should not overlook the beauty of the urban landscape.

The steel and glass of municipal mountains reflect the sunlight and make people feel small in the shadows. Birds sing in city parks, water burbles in the fountains, and along the sidewalks walkers can still see abundant wildlife—their fellow human beings.

Falcon's many outdoor guidebooks have encouraged people not only to explore and enjoy America's natural beauty but to preserve and protect it. Our cities also are meant to be enjoyed and explored, and their irreplaceable treasures need care and protection.

When travelers and walkers want to explore something that is inspirational and beautiful, we hope they will lace up their walking shoes and point their feet toward one of this country's many cities.

For there, along the walkways, they are sure to discover the excitement, history, beauty, and charm of urban America.

—*The Editors*

# Map Legend

| | | | |
|---|---|---|---|
| Walk Route | | Interstate | |
| Walk Route (boardwalk) | | State and County Roads | |
| Walk Route (bark) | | Start/Finish of Loop Walk | S/F |
| Streets and Roads | | Parking Area | P |
| Hiking/Walking Trail | | Body of Water | |
| Building | | Park/Open Space | |
| Restrooms, Male and Female | | Bridge | |
| Handicapped Access | | Church | |
| Picnic Area | | Interpretive Sign | |
| Playground | | Steps | |
| Tennis Courts | | Underground Bus Route | ••••• |
| Baseball Field | | Map Orientation | N |
| Stairs | | Scale of Distance | 0  0.5  1  Miles |

# Seattle Map Overview

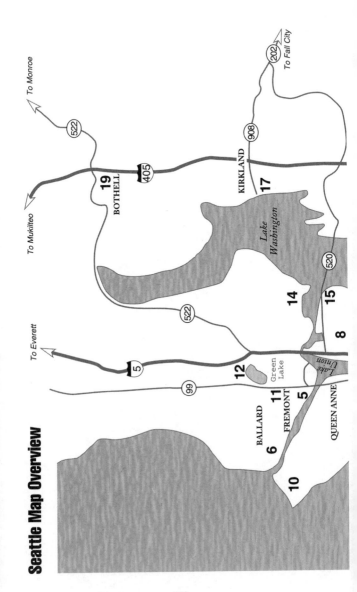

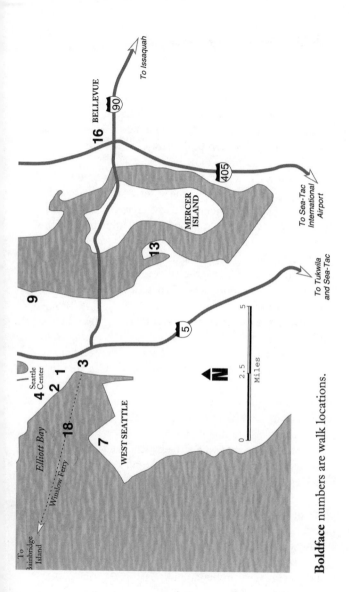

**Boldface** numbers are walk locations.

# Preface: Come Walk Seattle

Driving in Seattle is a hassle. Walking is a joy. Give the blame, or credit, to the lakes, oceanfront, and canals.

Seattle is flanked on one side by Elliott Bay and Puget Sound and on the other by Lake Washington. Then there are Lake Union, Green Lake, and numerous smaller lakes within the city that interrupt the flow of traffic but promote tranquility for travelers afoot.

The best walks in and around Seattle offer grand views or at least fleeting glimpses of the water. Seattle is also a city of hills, once covered thickly by native trees but now affording viewpoints from parks, parkways, and mini-parks within the residential communities.

It was not difficult to define the most rewarding walks in and around Seattle. The problem was limiting the choice from among 50 or more favorites described by people who reside in the various neighborhoods.

Much of the credit for these scenic routes should go to the New York firm of landscape architect Frederick Law Olmsted, which created Central Park for the residents of Manhattan. At the turn of the century, the Olmsted firm gave Seattle a master plan of community parks and greenbelts. It was ambitious and visionary, and it created an atmosphere of beauty and tranquility that residents have battled vigorously to maintain.

In contrast, downtown Seattle has changed dramatically in the past 100 years. A new art museum, a symphony hall, glittering new shopping plazas, two new sports stadiums, and several theater companies are all within walking distance of downtown offices and hotels. The city center is particularly vibrant at night, thanks to a thriving and continually changing restaurant scene.

So get out of your car, tighten the laces on your sneakers, and enjoy the City on the Sound.

# Introduction

Walking the streets and boulevards of a city can take you into its heart and give you a feel for its pulse and personality. From the sidewalk looking up, you can appreciate its architecture. From the sidewalk peeking in, you can find the quaint shops, local museums, and great eateries that give a city its charm and personality. From its nature paths, you can smell the flowers, glimpse the wildlife, gaze at a lake, or hear a creek gurgle. Only by walking can you get close enough to read the historical plaques and watch the people. When you walk a city, you get it all—adventure, scenery, local color, good exercise, and fun.

## How to use this guide

We have designed this book so that you can easily find the walks that match your interests, time, and energy level. The Trip Planner (see pages 8 and 9) is the first place you should look when deciding on a walk. This table will give you the basic information—a walk's distance, the estimated walking time, and the difficulty. The pictures or icons in the table also tell you specific things about the walk:

Every walk has something of interest, but this icon tells you that the route will have particular appeal to the shutterbug. So bring your camera. You will have great views of the city or the surrounding area, and you are likely to get some wonderful scenic shots.

Somewhere along the route you will have the chance to get food or a beverage. You will have to glance through the walk description to determine where and what kind of food and beverages are available. Walks that do not have the food icon probably are along nature trails or in noncommercial areas of the city.

1

During your walk you will have the chance to shop. More detailed descriptions of the types of stores you will find can be found in the actual walk description.

This walk features something kids will enjoy seeing or doing—a park, zoo, museum, or play equipment. In most cases the walks that carry this icon are short and follow an easy, fairly level path. You know your young walking companions best. If your children are patient walkers who do not tire easily, then feel free to choose walks that are longer and harder. In fact, depending on a child's age and energy, most children can do any of the walks in this book. The icon only notes those walks we think they will especially enjoy.

Your path will take you primarily through urban areas. Buildings, small city parks, and paved paths are what you will see and pass.

You will pass through a large park or walk in a natural setting where you can see and enjoy nature.

The wheelchair icon means that the path is fully accessible. This walk would be easy for someone pushing a wheelchair or stroller. We have made every attempt to follow a high standard for accessibility. The icon means there are curb cuts or ramps along the entire route, plus a wheelchair-accessible bathroom somewhere along the way. The path is mostly or entirely paved, and ramps and unpaved surfaces are clearly described. If you use a wheelchair and have the ability to negotiate curbs and dirt paths or to wheel for longer distances and on uneven surfaces, you may want to skim the directions for the walks that do not carry this symbol. You may find other walks you will enjoy. If in doubt, read the full text of the walk or call the contact source for guidance.

At the start of each walk description, you will find specific information describing the route and what you can expect on your walk:

**General location:** Here you will get the walk's general location in the city or within a specific area.

**Special attractions:** Look here to find the specific things you will pass. If this walk has museums, historic homes, restaurants, or wildlife, it will be noted here.

**Difficulty:** For this book we have selected walking routes that an average person in reasonable health can complete easily. In most cases, you will be walking on flat surfaces with few, if any, hills. Your path will most likely be a maintained surface of concrete, asphalt, wood or packed dirt. It will be easy to follow, and you will be only a block or so from a phone, other people or businesses. If the walk is less than a mile, you may be able to walk comfortably in street shoes. If you are in doubt about whether you can manage a particular walk, read the description carefully or call the listed contact for more information.

**Distance and estimated time:** This gives the total distance of the walk. The time allotted for each walk is based on walking time only, which we have calculated at about 30 minutes per mile, a slow pace. Most people have no trouble walking a mile in half an hour, and people with some walking experience often walk a 20-minute mile. If the walk includes museums, shops, or restaurants, you may want to add sightseeing time to the estimate.

**Services:** Here you will find out if such things as restrooms, parking, refreshments, or information centers are available and where you are likely to find them.

**Restrictions:** The most often noted restriction is pets, which almost always have to be leashed in a city. Most cities also have strict "pooper-scooper" laws, and they enforce them. But restrictions may also include the hours or days a museum or business is open, age requirements, or whether you can ride a bike on the path. If there is something you cannot do on this walk, it will be noted here.

**For more information:** Each walk includes at least one contact source for you to call for more information. If an agency or business is named as a contact, you will find its phone number and address in Appendix B. This appendix also includes contact information for any business or agency mentioned anywhere in the book.

**Getting started:** Here you will find specific directions to the starting point. Most walks are closed loops, which means they begin and end at the same point. Thus, you do not have to worry about finding your car or your way back to the bus stop when your walk is over.

In those cities with excellent transportation, such as Seattle, it may be easy—and sometimes even more interesting—to end a few of your walks away from the starting point. When this happens, you will get clear directions on how to take public transportation back to your starting point.

If a walk is not a closed loop, this section will tell you where the walk ends, and you will find the exact directions back to your starting point at the end of the walk's directions.

Some downtown walks can be started at any one of several hotels the walk passes. The directions will be for the main starting point, but this section will tell you if it is possible to pick up the walk at other locations. If you are staying at a downtown hotel, it is likely that a walk passes in front of or near your hotel's entrance.

**Public transportation:** Many cities have excellent transportation systems; others have limited services. If it is possible to take a bus or commuter train to the walk's starting point, you will find the bus or train noted here. You may also find some information about where the bus or train stops.

**Overview:** Every part of a city has a story. Here is where you will find the story or stories about the people, neighborhoods, and history connected to your walk.

# The walk

When you reach this point, you are ready to start walking. In this section you will find not only specific and detailed directions, but you will also learn more about the things you are passing. Those who want only the directions and none of the extras can find the straightforward directions by looking for the ➤.

**What to wear**

The best advice is to wear something comfortable. Leave behind anything that binds, pinches, rides up, falls down, slips off the shoulder, or comes undone. Otherwise, let common sense, the weather, and your own body tell you what to wear.

**What to take**

Be sure to take water. Strap a bottle to your fanny pack or tuck a small one in a pocket. If you are walking several miles with a dog, remember to take a small bowl so your pet can have a drink, too.

Carry some water even if you will be walking where refreshments are available. Several small sips taken throughout a walk are more effective than one large drink at the walk's end. Avoid drinks with caffeine or alcohol because they deplete rather than replenish your body's fluids.

**Safety and street savvy**

Mention a big city and many people immediately think of safety. Is it safe to walk there during the day? What about at night? Are there areas I should avoid?

You should use common sense whether you are walking in a small town or a big city, but safety does not have to be your overriding concern. American cities are enjoyable places, and you will find that they are generally safe places.

Any safety mishap in a large city is likely to involve petty theft or vandalism. So, the biggest tip is simple: Do not tempt thieves. Purses dangling on shoulder straps or slung over your arm, wallets peeking out of pockets, arms burdened with packages, valuables on the car seat—all of these things attract the pickpocket, purse snatcher, or thief. If you look like you could easily be relieved of your possessions, you may be.

Do not carry a purse. Put your money in a money belt or tuck your wallet into a deep side pocket of your pants or skirt or in a fanny pack that rides over your hip or stomach. Lock your valuables in the trunk of your car before you park and leave for your walk. Protect your camera by wearing the strap across your chest, not just over your shoulder. Better yet, put your camera in a backpack.

You also will feel safer if you remember the following:

- Be aware of your surroundings and the people near you.

- Avoid parks or other isolated places at night.

- Walk with others.

- Walk in well-lit and well-traveled areas.

The walks in this book were selected by people who had safety in mind. No walk will take you through a bad neighborhood or into an area of the city that is known to be dangerous. So relax and enjoy your walk.

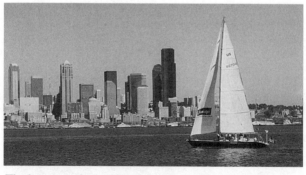

*The skyscrapers of central Seattle hug the shoreline of Elliott Bay.*

# Trip Planner

## the walks

| Walk name | Difficulty | Distance (miles) | Time | ♿ | 🏙 | 🌿 | 🎧 | 🔭 | 🐾 | 🛍 | 📷 |
|---|---|---|---|---|---|---|---|---|---|---|---|
| **Downtown** | | | | | | | | | | | |
| 1. City Center | easy | 2 mi | 1.5 hrs | | ✓ | | | | ✓✓✓ | ✓✓✓ | ✓✓✓ |
| 2. Pike Place Market | easy | 1.7 mi | 1 hr | | ✓ | | ✓✓ | | ✓✓✓ | ✓✓✓ | ✓✓✓ |
| 3. Pioneer Square | easy | 1.7 mi | 1 hr | | ✓ | | ✓✓ | | | | |
| **Neighborhoods** | | | | | | | | | | | |
| 4. Queen Anne Hill, Seattle Center | moderate | 4.5 mi | 2.5 hrs | | ✓ | ✓✓✓✓ | ✓✓✓✓ | ✓✓✓ | ✓✓✓ | ✓✓✓ | ✓✓✓✓ |
| 5. Fremont | easy | 3 mi | 1.5 hrs | | ✓ | ✓✓✓✓ | ✓✓✓✓ | ✓✓✓ | ✓✓✓ | ✓✓✓ | ✓✓✓ |
| 6. Ballard | moderate | 4 mi | 1.5 hrs | | ✓ | ✓✓✓✓ | ✓✓✓✓ | ✓✓ | ✓ | ✓ | ✓ |
| 7. West Seattle | easy/moderate | 5.7 mi | 2.5 hrs | ✓ | ✓ | ✓ | ✓ | ✓ | | | |
| **Parks** | | | | | | | | | | | |
| 8. Volunteer Park, Broadway District | easy | 2.5 mi | 1.5 hrs | | ✓ | ✓ | ✓ | ✓ | ✓✓ | ✓ | ✓ |
| 9. Madison Park | moderate | 4.7 mi | 2.5 hrs | | | ✓ | ✓ | ✓ | | | |
| 10. Discovery Park | moderate | 4 mi | 2.5 hrs | | | ✓ | ✓ | ✓ | ✓ | | ✓✓ |
| 11. Woodland Park Zoo | easy | 1.25 mi | 1.5 hrs | ✓ | | | ✓ | ✓ | ✓ | | |

| | | | |  Wheelchair access | City setting | Nature setting | Good for kids | Shopping | Food | Bring camera |
|---|---|---|---|---|---|---|---|---|---|---|
| 12. Green Lake | easy | 2.9 mi | 1.25 hrs | ✓ | | ✓ | ✓ | | ✓ | |
| 13. Seward Park (2 options) | easy/ moderate | 2.5 / 6.5 mi | 1.5 / 3 hrs | ✓ | | ✓ | ✓ | | ✓ | ✓ |
| **University of Washington** | | | | | | | | | | |
| 14. Campus | easy | 3 mi | 1.5 hrs | ✓ | | | | ✓ | ✓ | ✓ |
| 15. Washington Park Arboretum | moderate | 3 mi | 1.5 hrs | | | ✓ | | | ✓ | ✓ |
| **Suburbs** | | | | | | | | | | |
| 16. Mercer Slough Nature Park | easy | 2 mi | 1 hr | ✓ | | ✓ | | | ✓ | ✓ |
| 17. Kirkland | easy | 3.5 mi | 2 hrs | ✓ | | ✓ | | | ✓ | ✓ |
| 18. Bainbridge Ferry (2 options) | easy | 1.5 / 3 mi | 1.5 / 3 hrs | ✓ | | ✓ | | | ✓ | ✓ |
| 19. Sammamish River Trail | moderate | 7 mi | 3.5 hrs | ✓ | | ✓ | ✓ | | ✓ | ✓ |

**the icons**

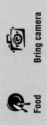

|  |  |  |  | | | |
|---|---|---|---|---|---|---|
| Wheelchair access | City setting | Nature setting | Good for kids | Shopping | Food | Bring camera |

## Meet Seattle

### General
County: King
Time zone: Pacific
Area code: 206

### Size
Washington's largest city
535,000 people within the city limits
3.1 million in metro area
84 square miles

### Elevation
10 feet above sea level

### Climate
Average annual precipitation: 38.2 inches
Average relative humidity: 74 percent (at 10 A.M.)
Average number of sunny days a year: 57.8
Average number of cloudy days a year: 225.6
Average number of partly cloudy days a year: 81.6
Average annual snowfall: 3.7 inches
Average maximum temperature: 60 degrees
Average minimum temperature: 46 degrees

### Major highways
Interstates: I-5, I-90, I-405
Washington State highways: WA 99, 509, 513, 520, 522, 523

### Ferry system
Washington State Ferry service to and from Bremerton, Vashon Island, Southworth, and Bainbridge Island; also from Edmonds to Kitsap Peninsula and from Mukilteo to Whidbey Island

### Airport service
Air Canada, Alaska, America West, American, British, Continental, Delta, Frontier, Horizon, Northwest, Reno,

Scandinavian, Southwest, Thai, Trans World, U.S., United

## Recreation

Bicycling: 30 miles of auto-free bike trails, 90 miles of signed bike routes

Golf courses in western Washington: 130 (114 public)

Hiking: Major areas include North Cascades National Park, Olympic National Park, Mount Rainier, Mount Baker, and along Snoqualmie Pass (I-90)

Number of parks: 406 city, 208 county

Saltwater fishing: 12 charter companies

Skiing: Six ski areas within 90 minutes of downtown Seattle

Boat rentals: Shilshole Marina, Lake Union, Green Lake, Seacrest Marina in West Seattle

## Major industries

Aircraft, computer and electronics, fishing, marine, shipbuilding, tourism

## Media

13 local television stations, including:

ABC—Channel 4

CBS—Channel 7

Fox—Channel 13

NBC—Channel 5

PBS—Channel 9

39 radio stations, including:

KIRO 710 AM—Talk and sports

KJR 950 AM—All sports

KING 98.1 FM—Classical music

KUOW 94.9 FM—National Public Radio member

KPLU 88.5 FM—National Public Radio member

Newspapers:

*Seattle Post-Intelligencer* (daily, morning)

*Seattle Times* (daily, morning)

## Special annual events

- January: Chinese New Year (call 206-623-8171), Seattle International Boat Show (206-296-3100)

- February: Northwest Flower and Garden Show (206-789-5333), Fat Tuesday (206-622-2563)

- March: Seattle Home Show (206-296-3100)

- May: Northwest Folklife Festival (206-684-7200), Seattle International Film Festival (206-324-9996), Yacht Parade (206-325-1000), Pike Place Market Festival (206-587-0351), University Street Fair (206-523-4272), Maritime Week on Puget Sound (206-443-3830)

- June: Edmonds Arts Festival (425-771-6412), Fremont Arts and Crafts Festival and Fremont Parade (206-632-1285)

- July: Fourth of July Fireworks (Myrtle Edwards and Gasworks Parks and several other locations), Pacific Northwest Arts and Crafts Festival (Bellevue, 425-454-4900), Bite of Seattle (206-232-2982), Chinatown Festival (206-725-1456)

- August: Seafair, including Torchlight Parade, Unlimited Hydroplane Races, community festivals (206-728-0123)

- September: Bumbershoot Festival (206-684-7200)

- October: Northwest Bookfest (206-378-1883)

- November: Harvest Festival (800-321-1213)

- December: Seattle Christmas Ships (206-461-5840), New Year's Eve at the Needle (206-443-2100), Winterfest (206-684-7200)

## Weather

Q—How do Seattle residents celebrate summer?

A—If it falls on a Sunday, they go on a picnic.

Q—What did Mark Twain say about Seattle's weather?

A—"The coldest winter I can remember was the summer I spent on Puget Sound."

Q—(Visitor to local boy) "Does it ever stop raining around here?"

A—"How should I know? I'm only six years old."

Forget the stereotype. Ignore the fact that one of the city's major celebrations—Bumbershoot—was given a slang name for umbrella. The fact is, Seattle ranks 44th among U.S. cities in annual rainfall. It does not rain as hard in Seattle as it does in Miami, New Orleans, or Chicago. However, it may rain longer in Seattle, because precipitation most often consists of prolonged drizzle. In any season, you should carry a small umbrella and a rain jacket in your daypack while walking.

Seattle residents normally experience only 57.8 cloud-free days a year. One of those days is likely to be July 30, when the odds are most favorable for sunshine and warm temperatures.

Seattle residents experience few days when the temperature tops 85 degrees F. Even when it does, the heat rarely carries over into the evening.

The winter lows are seldom extreme. Typically, less than an inch of snow falls at one time, and only occasionally does it remain on the ground for more than two days. Yet, you can find plenty of snow just an hour's drive from Seattle, at ski areas in the Cascades.

July and August are the hottest months, January and February are the coldest, and November and December are the wettest.

One other interesting fact: According to one survey, Seattle leads the nation in the sale of sunglasses per capita. Go figure.

## Transportation

**By car:** Traffic congestion in Seattle is among the worst in the United States, according to recent studies of urban communities. The traffic on I-5 during commuter hours in the morning and evening is especially heavy and should be avoided if possible. The same is true of the two floating-bridge routes, WA 520 and I-90.

There are a limited number of metered parking spaces in downtown Seattle, but overtime violations are costly. Parking lots and garages are numerous but also expensive during business and shopping hours.

Pay close attention to Seattle street signs and do not confuse Highland Drive (for example) with Highland Avenue, Highland Avenue South, East Highland Drive, West Highland Drive or Highland Lane.

I-5 runs through the center of Seattle and leads south to Portland and Tacoma and north to Everett, Bellingham, and Vancouver, British Columbia. Seattle street numbers increase as you travel north from the city's business district.

There are exits off I-5 to the communities east of Lake Washington. The I-90 exit off I-5 crosses a floating bridge to Mercer Island and South Bellevue. I-90 continues on to Snoqualmie Pass, Ellensburg, and Spokane. The WA 520 exit off I-5 crosses the Evergreen Point Floating Bridge to Kirkland and North Bellevue.

If you travel south on I-5 from downtown Seattle, an exit sign points the way to the bridge leading to West Seattle, the section of the city across Elliott Bay from the business district. Signs also indicate exits to the Washington State Ferry Terminal on the waterfront, the Washington State Convention and Trade Center in midtown, and the football-baseball stadium complexes just south of Pioneer Square.

Before I-5 was built, WA 99 was the main north-south thoroughfare. It is now marked as Aurora Avenue through much of Seattle.

**By bus:** The Metro Transit System is a wise alternative to driving, and bus travel is free within the main business and shopping district. This includes underground bus stations located along a tunnel that runs 20 blocks through downtown Seattle. The busiest station is beneath the Westlake Center shopping complex at Fifth and Pine Streets in downtown Seattle. Exact change is required for trips outside the free zone. Westlake Center is also a terminal for the monorail, which runs to the Seattle Center and back.

A trolley that runs along the Seattle waterfront and inland to Pioneer Square is part of the Metro Transit System. Community Transit operates buses from downtown Seattle north into Snohomish County. To the south, Metro Transit routes connect with service on the Pierce County Transit System.

An area-wide rapid transit project is under way and will eventually include both light and heavy rail, increased bus routes, and high-occupancy vehicle lanes.

Greyhound and Northwestern Trailways buses also operate out of Seattle.

**By air:** Sea-Tac International Airport is 13 miles south of Seattle. Ask for fare information before you accept a cab ride. The fare to or from downtown Seattle should be about $35. The Gray Line Airport Express offers bus service between the airport and downtown hotels for $7.50, or $13 round-trip. The Shuttle Express provides van service to and from hotels; it will also stop at residences and office buildings.

**By train:** Amtrak trains make daily runs from the King Street station south to Tacoma, Portland, San Francisco, and Los Angeles and north to Edmonds, Everett, Bellingham, and Vancouver, British Columbia.

## Safety

Downtown Seattle is considerably safer than many cities of comparable size, where workers flee to the suburbs when the sun begins to set. The restaurant and theater scene is vibrant. Shopping at Westlake Center, Pacific Place, and adjoining stores and malls continues well into the evening. More and more apartment and condominium towers are opening between the waterfront and business district and the business district and Seattle Center. There has been a corresponding increase in pedestrian traffic.

Some residents avoid the Pioneer Square area after dark because of the mix of street people headed for the missions and revelers attracted by the nightclub scene. Young people tend to congregate along Broadway and University Way. They occasionally ask passersby for spare change, but they are seldom threatening. Pike Place Market attracts a colorful mix of visitors and shoppers, which is part of the area's charm. Nonetheless, it is not a good place to loiter after dark.

Recreational walking is mainly a daytime activity, and the walks in this book are designed accordingly. None should be considered unsafe during daylight hours, but avoid walking in large, wooded city parks after dark. Lock valuables in the trunk of your parked car while you walk, and carry money in a fanny pack or daypack rather than in a purse or in a wallet tucked in a back pocket.

For a general review of city safety information, read the tips on pages 6 and 7. Enjoy your walks in this wonderful city.

# The Story of Seattle

When David Denny stepped ashore at the mouth of the Duwamish River in 1852, he might have been inclined to call the area Skunk Hollow, after some malodorous pests that promptly raided his meager food supply. Instead, his friend Lee Terry insisted that they name this future metropolis of the West after Terry's hometown of New York. The resident Indians expanded on the name with a word from the Chinook dialect, *alki*, which was loosely interpreted to mean "by and by." So the new settlement was known for a time as New York-Alki.

Within a few months, Denny and his party of pioneers decided that the site was not suitable for a permanent settlement, so they relocated across the bay. A land agent in Olympia identified their new settlement as Duwamps. The settlers quickly grasped for a new name. They decided to call their new home Seattle, after the Indian chief, Sealth, who welcomed them to the area.

Today Seattle is known variously as the City on the Sound and the Gateway to the Pacific Rim, while the Chamber of Commerce prefers the appellation Emerald City. It is also known as the home base for Boeing, Microsoft, Amazon.com, Starbucks, and Costco.

In the late 1800s, the city had another unofficial title. A census taken to create a tax base indicated that 10 percent of the residents were single women who lived within four blocks of Pioneer Square. They all described themselves as seamstresses, although they did not own a single sewing machine among them. Straight-faced city fathers created a $10-a-month "seamstress tax," and for the next five years, 87 percent of Seattle's operating funds came from this tax source.

So you might also describe Seattle as the Sewing Capital

of the Western World. And, as a matter of fact, a historical photo in the archives of a local industry shows 10 seamstresses affixing fabric to an aircraft wing. Thus was the Boeing Company launched in 1916.

But it was tall timber that created the first industrial base for the city. In 1792, the officers of the British ships *Discovery* and *Chatham* glimpsed the native forests along Puget Sound and speculated that there were enough trees to provide "masts and spars for all the navies of the world." This potential went unrealized until a treaty in 1846 established the boundaries of British and American holdings in the Pacific Northwest, encouraging an influx of settlers and speculators.

Denny, Terry, and John Low comprised the advance party for a group of 22 intrepid souls who arrived aboard the schooner *Exact* at what is now West Seattle. The soil proved unsuitable for farming, but there were trees aplenty. However, the anchorage proved too shallow to accommodate timber-hauling ships from San Francisco. So most of the settlers moved to a more suitable location across Elliott Bay.

The arrival of lumberman Henry Yesler, a native of Massillon, Ohio, jump-started Seattle's economy. Yesler built a sawmill after acquiring 320 acres of land along the waterfront from land speculators C.D. Boren and D.S. "Doc" Maynard. Yesler was able to hire just about everybody in the area who needed a job, including Chief Sealth. The timber shaped at Yesler's steam-operated mill provided the capital he needed to build the area's first hotel, bank, restaurant, post office, and water system. He served twice as Seattle's mayor.

When Yesler was 80, he wed a 20-year-old lass named Minnie Gagle who "lost" Yesler's last will and testament shortly after his death. Rumor had it that Yesler intended to leave $100,000 to the city of Seattle. Instead, Miss Minnie got the loot.

But Seattle survived. The city's development and growth were aided in no small measure by Doc Maynard, who had intended to join the California gold rush but was sidetracked to the Northwest. Maynard acquired thousands of acres in the new community. It was his idea to name the city Seattle. He surveyed, platted, and named many of the streets, and he served for a while as justice of the peace. The building that housed his business and general store was designated as the county seat.

But Maynard was a Democrat surrounded by Republicans, and he was a strong advocate of the Native American tribes, even after an Indian uprising in 1855. This skirmish between the settlers and Indians came to an abrupt end in 1856 after the arrival of the U.S. warship *Decatur* with a complement of Marines. But Maynard's status in Seattle suffered because of his loyalty to the tribes.

Two other figures who greatly shaped the future of Seattle were a woodworker and a newspaper editor. James McGough operated a paint and woodworking shop in the heart of the rapidly growing community. On June 6, 1889, his shop assistant allowed a glue pot to boil over onto a floor covered with turpentine and wood shavings. When McGough tossed a bucket of water onto the glue, he promoted, rather than prevented, a runaway fire. Despite the arrival of fire fighters, the flames spread to surrounding buildings. When whiskey barrels exploded in the basement of a nearby liquor store, the fire escalated into a full-scale disaster.

Within 12 hours, the entire business district and waterfront were gutted. Almost immediately, residents began to rebuild the central city. Tall brick buildings replaced the wooden stores, banks, and theaters. Streets were widened, and water and sewer services were improved.

At the time of the fire, Seattle's population was listed at 31,000. Less than a year later, it had grown to 37,000 and by 1900 it was 80,671. Ten years later, Seattle had 237,000 residents. Its growth was due in part to the Klondike gold rush and the efforts of local newspaperman Erastus Brainerd, who promoted Seattle as the gateway to the gold fields of Alaska. With the backing of the Chamber of Commerce, Brainerd wrote magazine and newspaper articles for publications across the land. He placed countless promotional ads, including a six-column layout in William Randolph Hearst's *New York Journal*. He mailed out 100,000 copies of a special edition of the *Seattle Post-Intelligencer*, to every postmaster, library, and newspaper in the country.

Bankers, builders, real estate agents, grocers, hardware suppliers, outfitters, and railroaders all reaped riches from the Klondike gold rush, and many returned to Seattle to enjoy their newfound prosperity. Seattle gained stature on the international scene, and this was reinforced by the Alaska-Yukon-Pacific Exposition of 1909. The exposition was staged on property owned by the University of Washington, and its legacy to the school was one of the most picturesque and impressive campuses in the country. President William Howard Taft and "The Great Commoner" William Jennings Bryant were among the 3.74 million visitors to the exposition.

By 1960, Seattle was booming. The Boeing Company employed half of all workers engaged in manufacturing in King County. City officials decided that another party was in order. The Century 21 Exposition, held in 1962, drew 9.6 million paying guests. The exposition grounds are still a center of entertainment and learning, showcasing the Space Needle, the Pacific Science Center, an opera house, a playhouse, a sports arena, and a ballet center.

Seattle today is, indeed, an Emerald City—not to be confused with New York-Alki, Duwamps, or Skunk Hollow.

*walk* 1

# City Center

**General location:** Downtown Seattle.

**Special attractions**: Walk-through waterfall, skyscrapers, interesting architecture, historic theaters, mini-park over freeway, tourist information office.

**Difficulty rating:** Easy; flat, almost entirely on paved sidewalks with curb cuts.

**Distance:** 2 miles.

**Estimated time:** 1.5 hours.

**Services:** Several restaurants, upscale urban malls, tourist information center, convention center, and shopping malls with accessible restrooms and drinking water.

**Restrictions:** Leash and scoop laws for pets enforced.

**For more information:** Contact the Seattle-King County Convention and Visitors Bureau.

# City Center

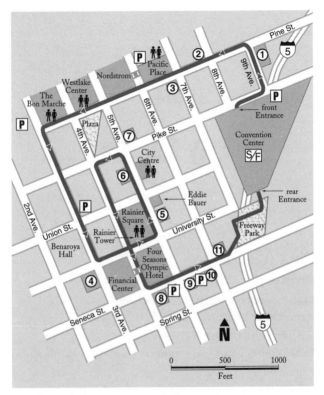

1. Paramount Theater
2. Paramount Hotel
3. Roosevelt Hotel
4. Washington Mutual Tower
5. Fifth Avenue Theater
6. Cavanaugh's Inn on Fifth Avenue
7. Coliseum Theater
8. Starwood W Hotel
9. YWCA
10. Crown Plaza
11. Park Place

**Getting started:** Take the Union Street exit off Interstate 5 Southbound to the first stoplight. Follow the sign that indicates an immediate right turn onto Seventh Avenue, and then make another right turn onto Pike Street. You can park in the Washington State Convention and Trade Center parking garage. The convention center, at 800 Pike Street, is a short walk from major downtown hotels.

**Public transportation:** Direct transportation is available on any bus route terminating or beginning in the Metro bus tunnel in downtown Seattle. Get off the bus at the convention center station in the tunnel.

**Overview:** Downtown Seattle is a work in progress, like a Broadway play, a symphony, or a major motion picture. In many American cities, the flight to the suburbs begins at 5 P.M., as the workday ends. To an encouraging degree, this trend has been reversed in Seattle. Suburbanites join downtown residents in the crowds attending sports events, concerts, plays, and movies. Or they participate in shopping excursions, art walks, and the vibrant restaurant scene.

This walk leads you through the areas of greatest change. Highlights include the new home of the Seattle Symphony, as well as theaters that were national showcases during the early years of the film industry and are now ageless treasures providing opulent settings for touring Broadway musical companies. Upscale shopping plazas, new hotels, and innovative restaurants are new jewels in the setting of downtown Seattle.

In 1907, the Moore Theater featured Sarah Bernhardt's film debut and a live appearance by the legendary actress. Nine years later, it screened Birth of a Nation, a silent-film epic accompanied by a live, 40-piece orchestra. The evening's entertainment included a parade of Civil War veterans from Seattle. In 1977, the Moore became the first home of the Seattle International Film Festival.

this downtown walk. So is the Coliseum, although it survives as a retail outlet and is no longer associated with the entertainment business.

The retail scene is a large part of the revival of downtown Seattle. And as a steel drummer performing in the plaza across from Westlake Center might observe, "It is all show business."

# the walk

Before starting the walk, you may wish to stop for maps and information at the Seattle-King County Convention and Visitors Bureau on the main floor of the Washington State Convention and Trade Center. A fountain inside the center marks the start of an escalator that serves four floors. Visitors are invited to tour the art exhibits on display on the third and fourth levels of the convention center.

➤Exit the convention center's main entrance on Pike Street to begin the walk.

➤Turn right immediately and walk up Pike Street beside the convention center for one block to Ninth Avenue.

➤Cross Pike Street and turn left onto Ninth. Note the New Orleans-style iron work and terra cotta designs on the sides of the large, red-brick Paramount Theater. Designed by B. Marcus Priteca, the Paramount opened in 1928 and was a showcase for vaudeville acts and major motion pictures. After the 1960s, it was used intermittently for rock concerts and an occasional closed-circuit telecast of boxing events. A multi-million-dollar restoration project, led by former Microsoft executive Ida Cole, saved the historic theater from the wrecking ball in 1995. Major Broadway-style shows are now presented in the Paramount.

➤Cross Pine Street and turn left. The theatrical name is

also attached to the recently renovated Paramount Hotel at Eighth and Pine.

Barnes and Noble is the first store you pass in the Pacific Place complex, starting at Seventh and Pine. Across Pine Street is the 20-story Roosevelt Hotel, the tallest hotel in town when it opened in 1930. It was recently renovated. Next door to the Roosevelt is Von's Grand City Café, which advertises itself as the "Martini-Manhattan Memorial."

Tiffany and Cartier are two of the more prominent names you will encounter when entering posh Pacific Place, which opened in 1998. Four restaurants and a multiplex theater occupy the fourth and top level. A sky bridge on the third level of Pacific Place allows shoppers to cross over Sixth Avenue to Nordstrom, which opened in 1901 as a local shoe store. The department store has since expanded into a nationwide chain but is still headquartered in Seattle. The block-square space between Fifth and Sixth Avenues was the longtime site of another major department store, Frederick and Nelson. When "F and N" closed, Nordstrom moved across Pine Street to the larger location, which was completely renovated in 1998.

Just past Nordstrom on Pine is Westlake Center, which was intended to be the center of Seattle's downtown retail-business district when the $250 million project was launched in 1988. Originally, Pine Street was closed to vehicular traffic in this block to create a plaza. Local retailers protested, and traffic was finally reintroduced.

A public plaza of more limited scope is just across Pine from Westlake Center. Here, musicians with panpipes and steel drums perform. A carousel lures children and their parents. An occasional civic rally for a local sports team draws the downtown crowds. But the plaza is probably most popular with people who simply sit and observe the passing parade.

Before you cross Fourth Avenue, note on your left the pedestrian-friendly waterfall. Bob Maki's stone and water sculpture was designed to be appreciated from the inside out. As you walk through it, you seem to be entering an elaborate shower stall. But unless the wind is particularly strong, you experience nothing more than a light misting—welcome relief during the occasional hot summer day.

Continuing on Pine, you pass the Bon Marché department store on your right. Plans for a multi-million-dollar renovation of "The Bon" were announced in 1998, just as Pacific Place and the new Nordstrom store opened.

➤Turn left onto Third Avenue. A fast-food complex on the left called the Rotunda features an indoor walkway connecting Third and Fourth Avenues.

➤Continue down Third and cross Pike Street. Third Avenue is experiencing a positive transition because of new developments like Benaroya Hall, home of the Seattle Symphony. The $118-million concert hall, which opened in 1998, takes up a full block between Union and University Streets.

Dale Chihuly's blown-glass chandeliers dominate the tri-level lobby of Benaroya Hall, designed by Mark Reddington and acoustician Cyril Harris. The hall features two concert spaces: the 2,500-seat Mark Taper Auditorium and the 540-seat Illsley Ball Nordstrom Recital Hall. The lobby is surrounded by glass, and the interior is lighted at night, casting a warm glow onto the streets outside.

Just inside the doors of Benaroya Hall on Third Avenue, fast-food booths serve members of the audience during concerts and are open to shoppers and local office workers during the day.

➤Turn left onto University Street, but note first the striking architecture of 55-story Washington Mutual Tower, with its foundation of pink Brazilian granite topped by patterns of faceted glass. The building dominates lower Third Avenue.

➤Walk uphill one block on University. On the four corners at Fourth and University are the downtown extensions of University Book Store, Alaska Airlines, the Four Seasons Olympic Hotel, and Rainier Tower, a curious high-rise that resembles a pencil stuck into the ground with the sharpened end down.

Rainier Tower was designed by Minoru Yamasaki, a Seattle native who also created the flowing arches of the Pacific Science Center beneath the Space Needle. Yamasaki also designed the World Trade Center in New York.

Between Fourth and Fifth on University, you pass the "coach entrance" of the Four Seasons Olympic Hotel. Built in 1924, the Olympic was Seattle's premier hotel for half a century. It was purchased and renovated by the Four Seasons chain in the 1980s.

➤Cross Fifth Avenue and turn left toward the marquee of the Fifth Avenue Theater, built in 1926. The interior, dominated by a dragon painted on the ceiling, was designed to resemble the throne room of Beijing's Forbidden City. The theater was restored in 1980 and now features touring companies of Broadway-style shows, as well as a celebrity lecture series.

To your left as you walk down Fifth Avenue are entrances to Rainier Tower and to Rainier Square, a complex of shops and restaurants that spans Fifth Avenue underground.

To your right at the corner of Fifth and Union Street is the showcase store of another homegrown company, Eddie Bauer, Inc. The namesake of the company was an avid hunter and angler who opened his first store featuring sporting equipment and outdoors wear in 1922. Eddie Bauer stores have recently expanded to all parts of the country, and the company is also a major catalog sales outlet.

To your left as you continue on Fifth Avenue past Union is yet another structure completed in 1998, Cavanaugh's Inn on Fifth Avenue. Directly across from Cavanaugh's is City Centre, a complex of upscale boutiques and shops. Located on the ground level of the high-rise U.S. Bank Center, City Centre is also the site of the popular Palomino Euro-Seattle Bistro.

Another classic Seattle theater, the Coliseum at Fifth and Pike, was converted in 1993 to a Banana Republic outlet. The interior design is unique for a retail store but offers only the barest hint of the theater's 1915 Italian Renaissance, terra cotta design.

➤Turn left onto Pike Street and proceed one block. The office-retail complex at Fourth and Pike with the large, circular windows is Century Square.

➤Turn left onto Fourth Avenue and walk past shops featuring jewelry and women's fashions and past the conference entrance to Cavanaugh's. The office buildings on both sides of the street reflect the unofficial height limits set by architects 40 and 50 years ago, before the high rises began to soar.

As you pass Union on Fourth Avenue you reach the main entrance to Rainier Square. At University Street you will have another view of the Four Seasons Olympic, including the skybridge from the hotel to the Financial Center. The office building and the rows of inset windows form a series of brown, rectangular blocks.

The Starwood W Hotel, across from the Four Seasons Olympic at Fourth and Seneca, open in 1999.

➤Turn left onto Seneca Street. Close to the "W" is the "Y"—the Downtown YWCA, that is, next to the Crown Plaza on Seneca.

**of interest**

### Whodunit?

It sometimes seems as though every fifth person you meet at a social gathering in Seattle is—or wants to be—a mystery writer. So it came as no surprise when a local travel agent, Connie Swanson, began offering an ocean "cruise with clues." Magnifying glasses, deerslayer hats, and gum shoes were not included. What the cruise did offer was a chance to meet and chat with J.A. Jance, author of the Beau Beaumont detective series.

The potential for this type of travel promotion is almost inexhaustible. Other tours could certainly be built around K.K. Beck, Earl Emerson, Valerie Wilcox, Richard Hoyt, or Mary Daheim, all of whom, like Jance, are residents of western Washington communities. It has been estimated that more than 30 crime writers live in or around Seattle, and they set many of their fictional scenes in familiar locations. There may soon be many more. Accompanying Jance on the first "clues cruise"—and available for consultation—was the author's literary agent.

Why does Seattle attract or produce so many real or aspiring mystery writers? One answer is obvious. "It was a dark and stormy night" describes a lot of evenings in western Washington. So the budding author has a lead sentence provided, free of charge.

Seattle also has a dark heritage. Serial killer Ted Bundy launched his crime spree in Seattle. The Green River Murders have never been solved. The Wah Mee Massacre claimed the lives of 13 residents of Seattle's Chinatown in 1983, and headlines pertaining to those crimes have appeared in Seattle newspapers ever since. Plus, crimes you never even imagined are detailed by a longtime Seattle private investigator, Windsor Olson, who loads curious residents and tourists into his van and gives them a grand tour of several nefarious sites. He performs this service whether the weather is dark and stormy or fair and mild.

➤At Seneca and Sixth Avenue, cross Sixth to the Park Place office building and the entrance to Freeway Park, a greenbelt built above the I-5 freeway through downtown Seattle.

➤Veer left just past Park Place and follow a sidewalk into the park. Concrete walls at the far end of the narrow park serve as waterfalls during summer months.

➤Walk to the waterfalls and the dedication plaques welcoming visitors to Freeway Park, which was opened on July 4, 1976, as part of the city's bicentennial celebration. To the left, you will see a low building fronted by green glass. That is the Washington State Convention and Trade Center, the starting and finishing point for this walk.

➤Turn left away from the plaques toward a staircase that leads out of the park, and climb the stairs.

➤Turn left onto the sidewalk at the top of the stairs. It heads toward the green convention complex. You will pass three flagpoles and enter the convention center's rear entrance.

*walk* **2**

# Pike Place Market

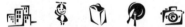

**General location:** On the waterfront, within walking distance of downtown hotels.

**Special attractions:** Victor Steinbrueck Park, produce vendors, fish merchants, arts and crafts vendors, specialty stores, restaurants, Bell Street Marina, the Seattle Aquarium, the Seattle Art Museum's Hammering Man sculpture.

**Difficulty rating:** Easy, with the exception of the climb from the waterfront to First Avenue via the Harbor Steps.

**Distance:** 1.7 miles.

**Time:** 1 hour.

**Services:** Dozens of restaurants and food stands in the market and along the waterfront, public restrooms in Pike Place Market and in the Seattle Aquarium building.

**Restrictions:** Leash and scoop laws for pets enforced.

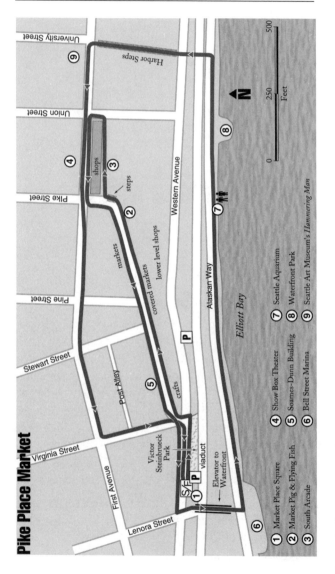

**Pike Place Market**

① Market Place Square
② Market Pig & Flying Fish
③ South Arcade
④ Show Box Theater
⑤ Soames-Dunn Building
⑥ Bell Street Marina
⑦ Seattle Aquarium
⑧ Waterfront Park
⑨ Seattle Art Museum's *Hammering Man*

Elliott Bay

N

0    250    500
Feet

**For more information:** Contact the Pike Place Market, Seattle Aquarium, or Seattle Art Museum.

**Getting started:** The market is within a short walk of most downtown hotels. Walk or drive west toward Elliott Bay on Pike, Pine, Stewart, or Virginia Street to reach the market. There is parking at the north end of the market along Western Avenue. This walk starts at Market Place Square, located at Western Avenue and Lenora Street above the main underground parking garage.

**Overview:** One of the great markets of the world, Pike Place Market is just a long grapefruit toss away from the heart of the hotel and financial center of the city. So this "walk" translates into an almost-daily luncheon stroll for a lot of downtown workers, shoppers, and visitors wearing Brooks Brothers suits, bib overalls, fashion pantsuits, or Seattle Mariner sweatshirts.

Not only can you smell the Pike Place Market from two blocks away, you can usually hear it as well. There are "ooohs," "ahhhs," and shouted warnings as onlookers watch a fish vendor scoop a 10-pound salmon off a bed of ice and send it spiraling like a football through the air to the counterman, who deftly catches it in an outspread sheet of wrapping paper. These are Seattle's famous "flying fish," but everybody associated with that scene would have been arrested under the original rules of order for the market. These rules, established in 1907, specified that:

- There will be no shouting of wares.

- Wagons full of produce must be parked at least five feet apart and backed into the curb.

- Wagons arriving first have their choice of locations.

- Farmer-merchants must arrive with their own refuse can in tow.

A Seattle police officer was dispatched to keep order on the morning of August 17, 1907, when the Pike Place Market opened to the public for the first time. Nobody really knew what to expect. A Renton farmer, H. O. Blanchard, was the first to pull into sight at dawn on that drizzly morning. Before he had a chance to back his wagon to the curb, waiting customers shoved the cop to one side and bought all the produce Blanchard had aboard.

Today the market is composed of concrete buildings, wooden sheds, a beehive of underground shops and stalls, rows of breathtaking blooms, and pyramids of Washington apples, radishes, onions, and melons. There are crumpet shops, French bakeries, and fishmongers selling Dungeness crabs and giant geoduck clams. There are posh restaurants, ethnic cafes, and stands selling fare from Mexico, Greece, Russia, and the Republic of Texas.

The Pike Place Market is no longer a simple hitching post for farm wagons. It is a complicated, clamorous, sometimes controversial citadel of cuisine, surrounded by luxury high-rise condominiums. It survived efforts in the 1950s and 1960s to either scrap it as an outdated and rat-infested relic or convert it into a glossy tourist mecca with an emphasis on hotel rooms and parking spaces.

In 1968, Mayor Dorm Braman described the market as "a decadent, somnolent fire-trap." But when world-renowned painter Mark Tobey returned to his hometown during this period of uncertainty he asked publicly, "What do we want? A world of impersonal modernism, a world of automobiles? I've studied and painted the Paris stalls, the markets of London, Mexico, and China and none is as interesting as ours. If anything should happen to the Market, I feel I would want to leave Seattle."

Tobey and Victor Steinbrueck, a University of Washington professor of architecture, goaded politicians and planners into bringing the market up to code without changing its essential flavor, image, or architecture. As a result, Seattle residents and visitors of today can still converge upon the Pike Place Market like smelt headed up the Columbia River during a spring run.

## the walk

The walk begins in Market Place Square, which is just above the Pike Place Market underground parking garage. Art galleries and a nature store dominate the square.

➤Head down Western Avenue in the direction of the central Seattle skyscrapers (east) and walk past Cutter's Restaurant and Victor Steinbrueck Park. The latter was named for the man who was instrumental in retaining a semblance of the original "Shop with the Producer" concept for Pike Place Market. Panhandlers, business executives, tourists, and local resident shoppers all congregate on the park lawn and benches to eat lunch on sunny days. The view, framed by totem poles created by James Bender, is of Elliott Bay and the container-ship terminals on Harbor Island.

Cars zoom along the Alaskan Way Viaduct below you, while ferries honk their way through small-boat traffic. You will probably spot an incoming freighter and an outgoing jet from Boeing Field or Sea-Tac International Airport.

➤Turn left at Virginia Street and cross Western Avenue.

➤Turn right and walk up the bay side of the market, past a long row of handicrafts peddled by or for local artisans. You will find paintings, glasswork, excellent photographs, pottery, jewelry, and games and clothes for kids.

The arts-and-craft theme continues as you pass under the market roof and head toward the distant displays of flowers, fruits, and vegetables. In the spring and summer, the flower displays on the low stalls to the left are spectacular.

You may want to take a detour once you reach the first fish market. If you want to spend 15 minutes or an hour roaming the countless shops in the underground portion of the market, head right, down the ramp. These lower-level shops sell everything from original King Kong posters to magic kits, herbs, coin and stamp collections, antique jewelry, and comic books. There is also a grocery store, a tiny barbershop, and a restaurant with a view "underneath" the market.

Otherwise, continue straight ahead toward produce row, also the location of a life-sized piggy bank, the "flying fish," and assorted street musicians. Tourists make an obligatory stop for a photo with or atop the "The Market Pig," but the biggest crowds are lured by the spectacle of animated fish vendors tossing silver salmon around like footballs.

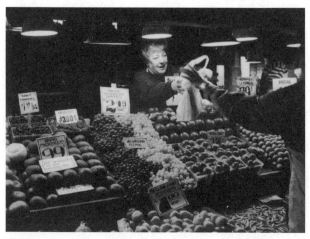

*Produce vendors at Pike Place Market feed thousands of shoppers every day.*

The Pike Place Fish Company may or may not be the best seafood shop in the market, but it is certainly the noisiest. Just beyond is Don and Joe's, one of the top meat markets in the city. The concourse turns left at a flower shop. If you follow the concourse to the street, you will pass DeLaurenti's Italian market, the Pike Place Art Stall, a fresh nut stand, a couple of food stalls, and the "Read All About It" newspaper and magazine stand, which carries periodicals from all parts of the country and world.

➤Our path makes a right turn at the back entrance to DeLaurenti's, at the sign that reads "Economy Market Atrium."

➤Walk down the staircase and continue straight ahead through the South Arcade. You will pass microbrewery tanks that draw attention to the restaurant one level below. Continue to the large picture window that allows you to watch the chefs at work in the kitchen of Leo Melina Ristorante Di Mare.

➤Execute a U-turn after you emerge from the market at First Avenue and Union Street. You will now head back up First Avenue, this time on the street side of some of the shops you have just passed. Across the street is the Show Box Theater. When it first opened, it was one of the first West Coast theaters to feature striptease "artiste" Sally Rand. After one block, you will again reach the "Read All About It" newsstand.

➤Walk straight across the street, with the light, toward Pike Place Flowers, and then turn left. On your right, note the sign for Crystal Market. You may want to explore some of these interior shops before continuing past the sign and following the traffic flow around the corner onto Pike Place. You will pass more fruit, cheese, seafood, and ice cream shops, as well as bakeries and ethnic fast-food stands.

**of interest**

### Hammering Man

He is silent, relentless, and ominous or hilarious, depending upon your point of view. But the thing that will most impress you when you confront him at the top of the Harbor Steps is that the Hammering Man is 48 feet tall. Described as the city's own $450,000 windup toy, he stands in front of—and identifies—the Seattle Art Museum.

According to Hammering Man's creator, Los Angeles artist Jonathan Borofsky, the sculpture is intended to represent workers everywhere, from farmers to aerospace engineers, from village craftsmen in Africa to computer operators in Seattle.

When most Seattle residents first became aware of the Hammering Man, he was lying face down at First Avenue and University Street. The 22,000-pound sculpture had crashed to the street when a nylon sling snapped during the first attempt to install the piece in 1991. Two years later, after the sculpture was finally in place, a group of local "art critics," whose spokesman identified himself as "Subculture Joe," affixed a 700-pound ball and chain to Hammering Man's ankle, in a tongue-in-cheek attempt to insure that he did not wander off. The deed was appropriately perpetrated on Labor Day.

Hammering Man made the local newspapers again in December 1996, when a group identified as the Hammering Santa Foundation placed a giant red and white knit cap on Hammering Man's head, purportedly utilizing a helium balloon to raise and adjust the Christmas "gift." Museum directors had to rent a telescopic boom crane so that Hammering Man could remove his hat.

Unshackled and bareheaded, Hammering Man continues to swing a sledge in front of the art museum, as do sim-
ilar Borofsky creations in Frankfurt, Germany, and Basel,
Switzerland. Borofsky has also created several smaller ver-
sions in his efforts to establish a "global village" of Hammering Men.

The Seattle Art Museum is open daily except Mondays. The Hammering Man never gets a day off.

to the Seattle Art Museum. The building was designed by
Robert Venturi and completed in 1991.

➤Turn left up First Avenue, where timid souls once feared
to tread. This area, once dominated by taverns and pawn
shops, is losing its rough-and-tumble reputation with the
addition of the art museum and the new Benaroya Hall.

➤Continue along First Avenue and pass the market entrance at Pike Street. Go straight past another row of interesting shops and restaurants on your left. They include the
Russian café Kaleenka and the venerable Virginia Inn,
known as an artists' hangout.

➤Turn left at Virginia Street and head downhill to Victor
Steinbrueck Park and the starting and finishing point of
this walk at Market Place Square.

*walk* 3

# Pioneer Square

**General location:** A 10-minute walk south of the business district, adjoining the waterfront.

**Special attractions:** Museum, several restaurants, interesting architecture.

**Difficulty rating:** Easy; flat, entirely on paved sidewalks.

**Distance:** 1.7 miles.

**Estimated time:** 1 hour.

**Services:** Klondike Gold Rush National Historic Park has water and restrooms.

**Restrictions:** Leash and scoop laws for pets enforced.

**For more information:** Contact the Seattle-King County Convention and Visitors Bureau or Klondike Gold Rush National Historic Park.

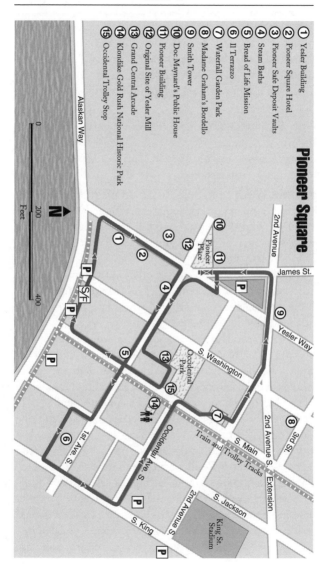

**Pioneer Square**

1. Yesler Building
2. Pioneer Square Hotel
3. Pioneer Safe Deposit Vaults
4. Steam Baths
5. Bread of Life Mission
6. Il Terrazzo
7. Waterfall Garden Park
8. Madame Graham's Bordello
9. Smith Tower
10. Doc Maynard's Public House
11. Pioneer Building
12. Original Site of Yesler Mill
13. Grand Central Arcade
14. Klondike Gold Rush National Historic Park
15. Occidental Trolley Stop

**Getting started:** From downtown Seattle, drive or walk to the waterfront, turn left onto Alaskan Way, and continue to the trolley station at South Washington Street. There are metered parking spaces underneath the Alaskan Way Viaduct. There are also several parking lots in the adjoining Pioneer Square area.

**Public transportation:** From downtown Seattle, walk to the waterfront. Board the southbound waterfront trolley at one of the mini-stations on Alaskan Way. Get off at the South Washington Street station.

**Overview:** Welcome to Skid Road, historic heart of Seattle, where the images of city founders Arthur Denny, Doctor Maynard, and the legendary Chief Sealth are recalled almost every step of the way around the district now known as Pioneer Square.

According to some historians, the land adjoining the Seattle waterfront was once a sacred rest camp for the Siwash Indians, who relished the salmonberries and clams that could be found here in abundance.

In 1852, the Denny party arrived at what is now West Seattle. After first wintering on Alki Beach, the settlers crossed the bay to relocate here and began to divide up the land. Maynard, another early settler, gave part of his land to Henry Yesler, who constructed a steam-powered lumber mill. Fallen trees were hauled—or skidded—down a steep slope to the mill. That route, now Yesler Way, was originally known as Skid Road. In a slightly altered form, this term spread across the country. Residents began to refer to rough-and-tumble neighborhoods in their cities as "Skid Row."

Seventeen years after members of the Denny party set up camp, Seattle was officially incorporated. By 1889, 40,000 residents were crowded into a jumble of wood-framed homes and stores. Most of these structures were destroyed by fire in June 6 of that year, when an overheated glue pot spilled in a furniture maker's shop.

The Pioneer Square area was rebuilt in stone and brick. After a steamship arrived in 1897 with news and hard evidence of the Klondike gold rush in Alaska, the area prospered. Prospectors bought their provisions in Seattle and then set sail from local docks.

By 1914, the Smith Tower, "the tallest building west of the Mississippi," loomed above Pioneer Square. Almost as soon as the area gained this prominence it began to lose it, as more and more businesses relocated to the north in what is now the commercial core of Seattle.

The creation of a historic preservation district in 1970 sparked the area's revival as an arts and crafts center, tourist mecca, restaurant district, and the gateway to another "gold rush" represented by millionaire athletes, multi-millionaire franchise owners, and the pleasure palaces that have recently been constructed to house Seattle's professional football and baseball teams.

# the walk

➤Facing Elliott Bay at the South Washington Street trolley station, turn right and walk one block on the pathway next to a railroad track.

➤Turn right onto Yesler Way and walk away from the bay. You are now entering the Pioneer Square district. The Old Yesler Building on the right is now the home of a popular Italian restaurant, Al Boccalino. Also on the right is the Pioneer Square Hotel, built at the turn of the 20th century and recently restored. Across the street is Trattoria Mitchelli, a popular and inexpensive pasta place. Just past Mitchelli on your left is a mini-storage sign in an alley; it marks the general area of the former Pioneer Safe Deposit Vaults, site of a Brinks-style robbery that took place in 1954.

➤Turn right at the intersection of First Avenue South and Yesler. The old Steam Baths sign marks the entrance to the Underground Seattle Tour. As you continue on First, you will pass a row of sidewalk cafés, specialty bookstores, art galleries, and imported-rug emporiums. The Bread of Life Mission, located at the intersection of First and South Main Street, is the site of Seattle's first store, built by Doc Maynard in 1890.

➤A block beyond the mission, cross South Jackson Street and turn right past the site of Seattle's first hardware company, built in 1905. Halfway down the block, turn left at a sign identifying a condo complex. This pathway will lead you to a picturesque mid-city retreat complete with waterfall, pool, and trees. You can enjoy a picnic here or join the diners inside at Il Terrazzo Carmine, a posh and popular Italian eatery named after the terrace it adjoins.

➤Continue straight ahead through the iron gates and immediately turn left onto South King Street. Sports souvenir shops and the headquarters of Seattle's major league teams reflect the proximity of this area to the twin stadiums built recently to replace the landmark Kingdome indoor arena.

➤Cross First Avenue South again and look down the alley on your left. You will get a good glimpse of the old Seattle, with its ivy-covered brick buildings, and the modern skyscrapers behind them.

The central hub of sports activity is F. X. McRory's, on your left at the intersection of South King Street and Occidental Avenue South. Mick McHugh and his former partner, Tim Firnstahl, opened McRory's in 1977. It was described then and remains today "a great joint" complete with the famed Whiskey Bar, which is reproduced in a Leroy Neiman painting that dominates the room.

➤As you turn left onto Occidental Avenue South, you can look through one of the large windows and glimpse McRory's bar and a display of some 150 different brands of whiskey offered inside. Straight ahead is a tree-lined pedestrian promenade that leads up to Occidental Park. The block just before the park is the center of the First Thursday Art Walks, which draw evening crowds to Pioneer Square each month.

➤Cross South Main Street and turn right. In a block you will reach Waterfall Garden Park, another mid-city gem. It was created in 1977 in memory of the deceased employees of the United Parcel Service. The company was founded here in 1907, and the site now features a waterfall that literally thunders down onto huge boulders, completely drowning out the usual sounds of the city.

➤Enjoy the park for a while and then exit through the far gate, turn left onto Second Avenue South, and head toward the Smith Tower. If you want to make a one-block detour to your right up South Washington Street, you will see a plaque on the building at Third and Washington identifying this spot as the former site of the Northwest's most famous and prosperous bordello, operated by Madame Lou Graham.

➤Continue on Second Avenue South, which becomes the Second Avenue South Extension as it leads to the Smith Tower. This historic landmark is still an impressive structure when viewed from street level looking straight up, but when viewed from an incoming ferry, it is dwarfed by recent construction. Built by L. C. Smith, of typewriter and armament fame, the 42-story tower was the fourth tallest building in the world when it opened on July 4, 1914. It is sheathed entirely in terra cotta and was designed by the Syracuse, New York, firm of Gaggin and Gaggin. Check with the elevator operator inside to see if the Smith Tower observation deck is open to visitors. If so, the deck offers dramatic views of Pioneer Square and the financial district.

➤Turn right onto Second Avenue South as you exit Smith Tower.

➤Turn left down James Street toward the waterfront. Off to your left you can glimpse the tower of King Street Station, from which trains head north to Vancouver, south to California, and east to Chicago.

A curious structure on your left has been nicknamed the "Sinking Ship Parking Garage," and you can easily see why. At the end of the block is Pioneer Place. There are totem poles, a bust of Chief Sealth, antique light fixtures, and the Pioneer Building, still a striking edifice representing the Romanesque style of architecture in Pioneer Square.

The Pioneer Building was built in 1889 on the site of Henry Yesler's first home. The structure was designed by Elmer Fisher, who designed more than 50 other buildings in the two years following the Great Fire of 1889. The Seattle Underground Tour begins at Doc Maynard's Public House, 610 First Avenue South.

Across the street from the Pioneer Building is a toy shop on the site of the original Yesler Mill.

➤From the Pioneer Building, retrace your steps up James Street to the crosswalk that takes you across James and Yesler Way to the Merchants' Cafe. The building was constructed just after the fire, in 1890. It became the Merchants' Exchange Saloon two years later and was owned by F. X. Shreiner, a member of a wealthy German family who sought adventure in the United States and found it serving with the U.S. Cavalry in the war against Geronimo.

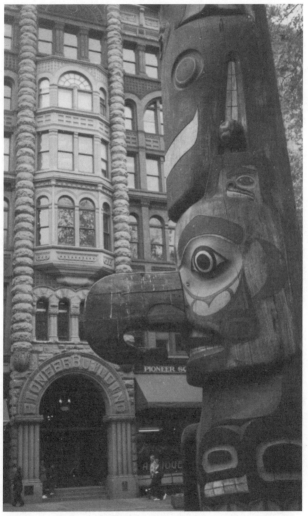

*A totem pole stands guard in front of the Pioneer Building, which was constructed just after the Great Fire of 1889.*

**of interest**

### Underground Seattle

Some tourists insist that the Seattle Underground Tour was the highlight of their trip to the city. Others wonder why they spent an hour or two of their vacation wandering in cellars, surrounded by crumbling bricks and weeping pipes. But both the critics and the enthusiasts agree that if you are genuinely interested in exploring in depth both the serious and humorous aspects of Seattle's history, the lectures delivered by Underground tour guides should fulfill that wish.

The Underground Tour begins at Doc Maynard's Public House, 610 First Avenue South, and lasts about 90 minutes. Included is a pre-walk lecture by a guide with lots of bathroom humor predicated on the fact that toilets once exploded upwards in Pioneer Square because of the sea-level location and the effect of the tides on a primitive sewage disposal system.

After the Great Fire of 1889 destroyed much of the original community, a unique plan for reconstruction was devised. It involved bringing in high-pressure hoses to wash down 200-foot cliffs, raising the elevation of Pioneer Square up to 10 feet above sea level. By the time this project was completed and new sidewalks laid, many business had already been rebuilt over the fire rubble, at the original street level.

Residents shopped in these basement-level locations from 1892 until 1907, when bubonic plague threatened the city. Officials took several steps to help prevent the spread of the disease, one of which was to require residents to carry a gun whenever they visited the outhouse, in case they encountered a rat. Under another new law, the underground buildings were sealed with cement. New stores were built above them.

When the threat of disease diminished, Underground Seattle briefly reopened as a site for speakeasies, gambling parlors, and bordellos. During World War II, officials shut down this "sin city."

These stores and corridors were empty for several years before a local author, historian, and promoter named Bill Speidel conceived the idea of running organized tours through the buried historical sites. The first tours were offered in 1965.

The 30-foot standup bar in the Merchants' Cafe was transported by schooner around Cape Horn near the turn of the 20th century. Hooks on the outside walls of the building were used to lower beer kegs into basement wells. During the Depression, the Merchants' Cafe served five-cent beers with free sandwiches and hardboiled eggs.

➤Walk half a block toward the waterfront along Yesler Way and then turn left onto First Avenue South. As the sign indicates, the old State Hotel once offered 75-cent rooms.

As you continue down First, you will pass several interesting shops and restaurants before reaching and entering the Grand Central Arcade, which has shops on two levels. The structure was built in 1890, and it served for a time as the Grand Central Hotel and then Squire's Opera House, the first performance theater in Seattle. For a few years, it was a glorified flophouse; then it was one of the first structures renovated during the start of the Pioneer Square revival. Good soup and sandwiches are available inside the Arcade. The shops in the basement occupy what was once the street level of early Seattle, before this district was raised out of the mud banks.

➤Exit the Grand Central Arcade through the back door, into Occidental Park. Immediately turn right and take the crosswalk across South Main Street to the building identified as the Klondike Gold Rush National Historic Park. This storefront museum features films, displays, and literature reliving the colorful era when Seattle was a gateway to the Alaskan gold fields. After deaths and near-disasters among the miners participating in the rush, the government began to require each prospector leaving a port like Skagway to buy and carry at least one ton of supplies in order to enter the gold fields. In the center of the museum, a display shows just how much food that was.

➤Turn left as you exit the Klondike exhibit and proceed to Elliott Bay Books, where many of the world's top contemporary authors have read from their works. Elliott Bay is one of the biggest independent bookstores in the West. If you need a break, there is a café in the basement, which gives you another chance to "visit" Underground Seattle. The frequently packed lecture area is also on the lower level.

➤If you decide to spend another hour or three in Pioneer Square, pick up the free newspaper, Discovering Pioneer Square. There should be a stack of them just inside the doorway of Elliott Bay Books. If you are leaving the area, you can catch the trolley at the Occidental Park station just in front of the Klondike exhibit. Or walk down South Main Street to the waterfront and Pier 48.

➤When you reach Alaskan Way on South Main, turn right and go one block to the South Washington Street trolley station and the starting and finishing point of this walk.

## *walk* 4

# Queen Anne Hill and Seattle Center

**General location:** About a mile northwest of the city center.

**Special attractions:** Space Needle, Seattle Center amusement park, Pacific Science Pavilion, International Fountain, Center House Food Circus, views of Seattle, historic homes, mini-parks, and a lively shopping-café district.

**Difficulty rating:** Moderate; almost entirely on sidewalks, but route includes steep grades and staircases.

**Distance:** 4.5 miles.

**Estimated time:** 2.5 hours.

**Services:** Restaurants, restrooms.

**Restrictions:** Dogs must be leashed and their droppings picked up.

# Queen Anne Hill and Seattle Center

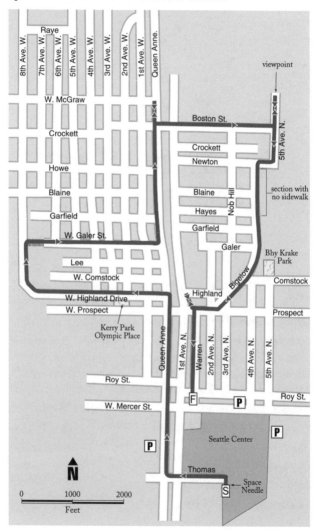

**For more information:** Call the Seattle-King County Convention and Visitors Bureau or the Queen Anne Chamber of Commerce.

**Getting started:** This walk starts at the Seattle Center, just beneath the Space Needle, which is visible from downtown. The easiest way to reach the center from the downtown hotels is via monorail, which leaves from Westlake Center. If you are driving, take the Mercer Street exit from Interstate 5 and follow signs leading to the Seattle Center. There are parking garages and lots on all sides of the center.

**Public transportation:** The best way to reach the Seattle Center is via the monorail from Westlake Center, 400 Pine Street. You can also take Metro Transit Bus 3, 4, 6, or 16 traveling northbound on Third Avenue in downtown Seattle for the short ride to the Space Needle. Check with Metro Transit customer assistance for bus stop locations and times.

**Overview:** The Space Needle was considered innovative architecture when it was built for Seattle's Century 21 Exposition in 1962. The name did not reassure nearby residents when construction began. A "needle" of steel was somehow going to provide balance and support for a sky-high observation deck and a revolving restaurant. Skeptics writing to local newspapers suggested that the structure would topple like a giant Northwest fir when the first storm swept off nearby Elliott Bay. The resultant crash, it was said, would shake foundations and shatter windows from Anchorage to Acapulco.

On opening day of the "World's Fair" in 1962, many of these doubters preferred to let tourists fill the elevators for the first few trips up the Needle. When the visitors survived the experience, the rush was on, and virtually all of the 10 million fairgoers made at least one trip to the top for a rubberneck survey of the city.

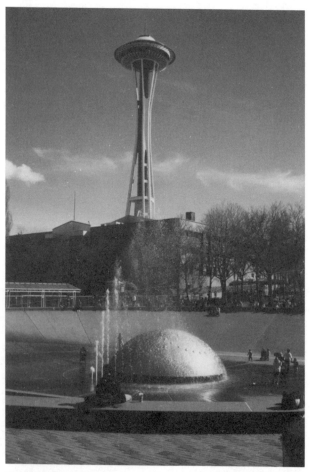

*The Space Needle looms over the Seattle Center, a legacy of the Century 21 Exposition, held in 1962.*

This walk gives present-day visitors a close-up look at the Space Needle and all the other attractions on the Seattle Center grounds. It also offers a long-range view from nearby Queen Anne Hill.

The 74-acre park known as Seattle Center is the city's most visible legacy from the Century 21 Exposition. When the fair opened, visitors scurried around the grounds inspecting dynamos from Russia and ancient pottery from Peru. They peeked at scantily clad dancers in Gracie Hansen's Paradise International and saw grand opera and the Old Vic Players on newly erected stages. Expo promoters invited the fan who caught Roger Maris's record-breaking home-run ball to come to Seattle and try to snag a horsehide dropped from the Fun Forest Ferris Wheel. (He failed.) Chickens tried to earn kernels of corn by pecking out codes in the Science Pavilion.

The graceful arches of the original science pavilion remain, but the building has been renovated and enlarged. The Food Circus has been remodeled and renamed Center House, but it still offers quick snacks or full meals representing the cuisine of 20 or 30 nations. Microsoft millionaire Paul Allen has financed construction of a new rock-and-pop music hall of fame. The amusement park now features the latest rides. Seattle Center provides a home for Pacific Northwest Ballet and four theater companies, plus the Seattle Totems hockey team, the Seattle Sounders soccer club, and the Seattle Sonics of the National Basketball Association.

The grounds are jammed each Memorial Day weekend for the Northwest Folklife Festival and again over Labor Day for Seattle's colorful Bumbershoot celebration.

You can spot most of the Seattle Center landmarks from several viewpoints atop Queen Anne Hill. Many times you will turn a corner and find yourself looking head-on at the observation deck of the Space Needle.

You can explore the Seattle Center grounds before or after this walk. A trip to the top of the Space Needle is almost obligatory—and, yes, it is safe. That was reaffirmed a couple of decades after the Needle opened to the public. At the same moment that a teeth-rattling earthquake shook Seattle, the original architect of the Space Needle just happened to be eating breakfast in the revolving restaurant at its top. Not once did he glance around for an exit sign.

## the walk

➤The walk starts at the base of the Space Needle. From there, head past the Center House. You will pass the Seattle Children's Theater on your left. This will take you out of the Seattle Center grounds on Thomas Avenue.

➤Turn right onto Queen Anne Avenue North. You will pass bakeries, espresso stands, and some excellent restaurants in the lower Queen Anne District.

There was once a cableman's shack on Queen Anne North where you begin to climb uphill. This was the route of a San Francisco-style trolley, which carried passengers to the top with the aid of a counterbalance. A flatcar passed downhill through an underground tunnel while the trolley headed up. Seattle's cable-car fleet was dismantled shortly before World War II.

➤At the fork at the bottom of the hill, go straight and up the steepest portion. The condominiums on your left on Queen Anne Avenue were once the frequent target of a cat burglar, whom local residents called Spider Man. Using ropes and grappling hooks, he scaled the side of the buildings to reach decks or sliding windows. Spider Man was blamed for at least 14 burglaries before a suspect was arrested in 1986. The suspect escaped conviction but the burglaries stopped.

➤Continue up the hill and then turn left onto West Highland Drive. Whitney Treat, a business associate of John D. Rockefeller, built the "House of Fourteen Gables" at 1 West Highland Drive for $100,000. The mansion housed Treat's family of four, plus 14 servants. On one occasion, Treat brought Buffalo Bill Cody and his Wild West troupe to Queen Anne to entertain his daughter on her ninth birthday. In the 1970s, "Gable House" was converted into 15 private apartments.

As you continue on West Highland Drive, you reach Kerry Park on your left. One glance tells you why this is the camera position of choice when network news crews come to Seattle. The view encompasses downtown Seattle, the Space Needle, Seattle Center, and—on a clear day—Mount Rainier in the distance. Also witness the marine traffic on Elliott Bay. Chances are you will see a ship tied up at the grain elevators. Noodle makers throughout the Orient prefer the wheat exported from this terminal.

Across the street from Kerry Park, at 222 West Highland Drive, is a house designed by an architect who worked out of Frank Lloyd Wright's offices. The mansion at 405 West Highland once housed the Japanese consulate.

You will pass several more million-dollar homes with two-million-dollar views. Note on the north side of West Highland Drive the lovely mini-park known as Parsons' Gardens, an urban hideaway popular for weddings. Across the street from Parsons' Gardens is yet another marine viewpoint. This one features stone sculptures by artists who are now legendary in Seattle, including Mark Tobey, Kenneth Callahan, Morris Graves, and Guy Anderson. There is also a granite sculpture by James Washington, Jr. This site is dedicated to the late Betty Bowen, an avid supporter of Northwest arts.

➤The path curves to the right along a walkway featuring light globes every 20 yards. Turn right at the West Galer Street sign and climb 77 stone steps. You are now near the top of Queen Anne Hill. Continue straight ahead on West Galer. In front of you are television towers, which are festooned with Christmas lights during the holiday season.

At 515 West Galer, you pass the old West Queen Anne Elementary School, built in 1896 and since converted to condominiums.

➤Turn left onto Queen Anne Avenue North. You will pass though a bustling community featuring coffee shops, bakeries, grocery stores, and several ethnic restaurants.

➤Continue up to West McGraw Avenue and check out A and J Meats, possibly the best and most complete meat market in Seattle.

➤Cross Queen Anne and double back one block to Boston Street.

➤Turn left onto Boston and continue all the way to Fifth Avenue North.

➤Turn left onto a dead-end road to a viewpoint overlooking the University of Washington campus and Lake Union. Note Gasworks Park on Lake Union, which you can identify by its giant, abandoned boilers. The Lake Washington Ship Canal passes Husky Stadium, through the Montlake Canal to Lake Washington. A boat traveling the waterway in the opposite direction could eventually reach China, via the locks at Ballard.

➤Turn around and head back down Fifth Avenue North, past a succession of architecturally unique but uniformly expensive homes.

### Queen Anne Hill

In the 1850s, native trees covered Queen Anne Hill. Below was Potlatch Meadows, tended by members of the Duwamish tribe. The Seattle Center now occupies the meadow site.

When houses began to replace the trees on Queen Anne, residents rode up something called the "Counterbalance" in a rattling cable car. As each car approached the hill, a worker attached a cable. At the opposite end was a flat rail car, which rode on separate tracks built beneath Queen Anne Avenue. This provided the counterbalance for the passenger cars.

The Queen Anne District features a dozen city parks, miles of boulevards, and more than 100 public staircases.

At one time, West Highland Drive, at the top of the hill, was the most prestigious address in Seattle. Alden J. Blethen, founder of the Seattle Times, was among the people who lived there. He volunteered to pay personally for the nightly lighting of gas lamps along the length of Highland Drive.

However, some longtime residents insist that Queen Anne Hill's most famous resident was Rocky the Rooster. According to private investigator Windsor Olson, who lived for several years on the hill, three roosters and 18 hens materialized one day on the hillside on Third Avenue North. Where they came from, nobody knew. But it became apparent that they were not inclined to soon depart. The roosters' nighttime crowing began to drive the residents up the native trees. So a plan was hatched to spike some chicken feed with vodka and then merely hand-gather the cross-eyed cluckers. The chickens developed a taste for the vodka, but imbibed in moderation.

Soon the residents resorted to pellet guns and medicated darts, but when they shattered a few windows and pocked some of the stonework, a cease-fire was called. By that time, both animal welfare organizations and local TV crews were fully alerted. So when someone decided to chase the chickens—and TV cameramen—down the street with salmon nets, the scene soon resembled an outtake from a Marx Brothers comedy.

Olson says most of the chickens died natural deaths after living out their lives on Queen Anne Hill. Rocky was the last to go, and his passing was marked by an obituary in the Seattle Times.

➤Turn right onto Newton Street and then left onto Bigelow. There are no sidewalks for the next couple of blocks, so walk on the left facing what little traffic you will encounter. After the sidewalk resumes, you will pass through the largest grove of European chestnut trees west of the Mississippi.

➤Take a half-block detour left onto Comstock Place to a viewpoint known as Bhy Krake Park. It looks down on the heart of the skyscraper district of downtown Seattle.

➤Return up Comstock and turn left again onto Bigelow, which becomes Prospect Street.

➤Bearing right on Prospect, you will come to a large building at First and Highland. This is the new Japanese consulate, located in the former C. D. Stimson mansion, built in 1898.

Look for the yellow house at the top of the hill. Legend says it once belonged to a bootlegger who used lanterns in the windows to send signals to his boats in Elliott Bay.

➤Turn around, retrace your steps back to Warren Avenue, and turn right, down the hill. Via the street and two stairways, you will return to the lower Queen Anne area past Larry's, one of the city's biggest supermarkets. You will spot Key Arena and the Space Needle looming just ahead, completing your loop walk.

*walk* 5

# Fremont

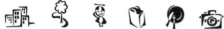

**General location:** Just north of Lake Union, approximately 3 miles from downtown Seattle.

**Special attractions:** Gasworks Park, overlooking Lake Union and the Seattle skyline; the Lake Washington Ship Canal; and the community of Fremont, Seattle's "Little Bohemia."

**Difficulty rating:** Easy; sidewalks and a few paths, with no elevation gain except for a steep uphill grade on the side trip to the Fremont Troll.

**Distance:** 3 miles.

**Estimated time:** 1.5 hours.

**Services:** Restrooms and picnic areas at Gasworks Park; several restaurants in the Fremont business district.

**Restrictions:** Leash and scoop laws for pets enforced.

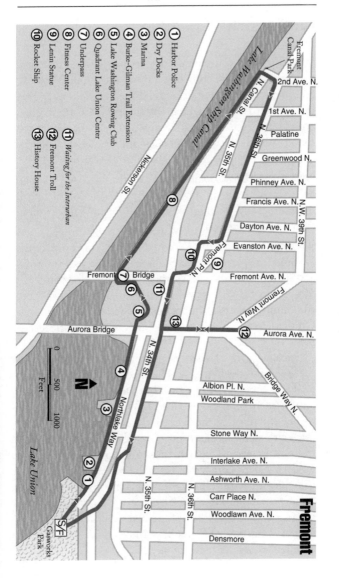

① Harbor Police
② Dry Docks
③ Marina
④ Burke-Gilman Trail Extension
⑤ Lake Washington Rowing Club
⑥ Quadrant Lake Union Center
⑦ Underpass
⑧ Fitness Center
⑨ Lenin Statue
⑩ Rocket Ship
⑪ *Waiting for the Interurban*
⑫ Fremont Troll
⑬ History House

Lake Washington Ship Canal

Fremont Canal Park

2nd Ave. N.
1st Ave. N.
Palatine
Greenwood N.
Phinney Ave. N.
Francis Ave. N.
Dayton Ave. N.
Evanston Ave. N.
Fremont Ave. N.
Fremont Way N.
Aurora Ave. N.

N. Canal St.
N. 36th St.
N. 35th St.
Fremont Pl. N.

Fremont Bridge

Aurora Bridge

Nickerson St.

N. 34th St.
Northlake Way

Albion Pl. N.
Woodland Park
Stone Way N.
Interlake Ave. N.
Ashworth Ave. N.
Carr Place N.
Woodlawn Ave. N.
Densmore

N. 35th St.
N. 36th St.

Bridge Way N.

N. W. 39th St.

**N** ▲
0 — 500 — 1000 Feet

Lake Union

Gasworks Park
SF

**Fremont**

**For more information:** Contact the Fremont Chamber of Commerce.

**Getting started:** The walk starts at Gasworks Park, at the north end of Lake Union. From downtown Seattle, take Westlake Avenue north around the lake and then go right onto Fremont Avenue and the Fremont Bridge. Turn right again onto North 34th Street and proceed to the park, which you can identify by the looming boilers and machinery from the abandoned city power plant. Parking at Gasworks is free.

**Public transportation:** Board Metro Transit Bus 26 northbound on Fourth Avenue in downtown Seattle. Get off at North 35th Street and Wallingford Avenue North. Walk downhill three blocks to the park.

**Overview:** What do the Wright Brothers, Vladimir Ilyich Lenin, Pearl Jam rock star Stone Gossard, a two-ton troll, and "rocket scientist Dr. Werner Von Hoge" have in common? They are all closely identified with Fremont, a Seattle community that has adopted as its civic slogan Delibertas Quirkas!, which locals translate as "Freedom to Be Peculiar."

Peculiar? Civic leaders have proclaimed Fremont to be the Center of the Universe. The exact spot is occupied by a 53-foot rocket, built in Korea but brought to Fremont by local resident John Hogh (alias Dr. Werner Von Hoge). The rocket is perched in the heart of the community, near a heroic-sized statue of Lenin and only a short rocket burst away from the Fremont Troll, two tons of reinforced concrete that lurks in a dark corner not far from a music studio established by Gossard. Oh, yeah, the Wright Brothers of Fremont repair bicycles, not airplanes. This would not be peculiar except that some of the bikes they repair have appeared in the annual Fremont Solstice Parade, mounted by members of a sometimes-nude drill team.

This walk passes through the old section of Fremont, with its wall-to-wall curio shops, ethnic restaurants, art galleries, and blue-collar taverns. It also passes through the new Fremont, with its luxury apartments and the recently built Adobe Systems computer software complex lining the ship canal.

Will the "Invasion of the Computer People" change the "hip" image and personality of Fremont? After all, this is a community where, on summer evenings, residents don costumes and carry their deck chairs, inflatable pads, and communal sofas "downtown" to watch movies on an outdoor screen.

The change is not obvious yet. Signs in Fremont still read, "Caution. Adults at Play." Chocolate "troll toes" are still the candy of choice. The community is still putting up "hysterical markers," like the one that claims "Fremont is sitting on top of a huge natural reservoir holding the largest proven beer reserves in the world."

Fremont does, in fact, sponsor a Beer Trek among three resident breweries: Redhook, Hale's, and Dad Watson's. There is also a lively Sunday street market and a First Saturday Art Walk. Fremont has 15 art galleries, the Empty Space theater company, and some 40 restaurants and/or pubs.

Fremont also has a history. There were a lumber mill and a few outbuildings in the area in the 1880s. By 1891, there were 5,000 residents in the area fed by one rail line. The community's front door, the Fremont Bridge, was built in 1916 after the construction of the ship canal linking Lake Washington and Lake Union with Puget Sound.

## the walk

➤From the parking lot of Gasworks Park, walk to the path at the foot of the hill and follow it away from the steam towers and boilers. The hill and Lake Union will be on your left. The path soon leads onto a traffic-free surfaced road. On your left are the boat docks for the Seattle harbor police. Just beyond them are the commercial ship docks and dry docks. You can usually spot several large crab boats, their decks stacked with traps and large orange floats.

►Stay on the left side of the road. At this point the sidewalk alternates with a dirt path. At a wide viewing area, you can inspect the fleet and watch workers repair boats. Looming straight ahead of you as you continue the walk is the Aurora Bridge, a high span over the canal leading out to Puget Sound. The commercial shipping scene on your left soon gives way to moorage for sailboats and pleasure cruisers. There is also a great view of the Seattle skyline.

►Stay on a path that is on the left side of a traffic guard. When you reach a sign reading "Waterway No. 22," cross the unmarked road to your right, but do not cross busy North 34th Street. Take the pedestrian pathway on the left side of the long brick building, which houses a restaurant. You are now on a section of the Burke-Gilman Trail, a former railway right-of-way that is now a heavily used, paved hiking and bicycling path.

The large building ahead of you that looks like a railway depot actually houses the shells and offices of the Lake Washington Rowing Club. You will pass to the right of this structure, and the path will lead you through the recently constructed Quadrant Lake Union Center and the local headquarters for the Adobe Systems computer software company.

►Remain on the Burke-Gilman Trail as it turns left and then passes over an unmarked road at a painted crosswalk. To your left are some small-boat moorages and a segment of Seattle's houseboat community. At this point the Aurora Bridge is directly overhead. The trail continues down to the water, where two picnic tables are located next to a Lake Washington Rowing Club dock.

➤Stay on the Burke-Gilman Trail as it turns right. You will pass between the Lake Washington Ship Canal and the Adobe complex.

➤Continue to follow the marked path as it leads you under the Fremont Bridge and passes between two warehouses. This is a work area frequented by trucks and forklifts, so proceed with caution. The pedestrian and bicycle path is clearly marked on the asphalt.

When the path leaves the warehouse area, the ship canal will be on your left. This portion of the canal links Lake Union with the locks at Ballard and with Puget Sound.

On the right of the pathway is a large building housing the Sound Mind and Body Fitness Center. Just past this structure, the path continues straight ahead along a tree-lined boulevard. Signs along the sidewalk indicate that one side of the path is designated for walkers, and the other side is reserved for bicyclists and skaters.

On your right at Canal Street and Phinney Avenue North is the Redhook Ale Brewery, which serves lunch. Farther along, on the other side of the canal, are the athletic fields of Seattle Pacific University. The campus stretches a couple of blocks inland from the canal.

Viewing and picnicking benches along the canal path offer you the opportunity to inspect the passing nautical parade of working and recreational boats. The biggest and last viewing area on this stretch is Fremont Canal Park.

➤The trail continues straight ahead, but we turn right at the park. Walk up to the intersection of North 36th Street and Second Avenue North. At this intersection, turn right and take the sidewalk along North 36th. Note across the street the George and Dragon Pub, a bit of old England crammed between aging buildings.

After a couple of blocks, you begin to glimpse the Fremont scene. Without altering your path, you will have the opportunity to get an acupuncture treatment, hear a lecture on Chinese herbal medicine, or get a $10 "buzz" haircut. You can buy a mandolin, a Japanese bento box lunch, a cinnamon roll, a pair of used snowshoes, dog biscuits shaped like poodles, or a tattoo.

At the intersection of Evanston Avenue North and Fremont Place North is the heroic-sized statue of Lenin.

►At Evanston, turn right and head back toward the canal. Ahead of you is a rocket ship, seemingly ready for takeoff. According to Fremont residents—who say they base their theory on Indian legend—the rocket ship is located at the exact center of the universe.

►Turn left onto North 35th Street to read the plaque at this official Fremont "hysterical site." It explains the significance of the space-age totem. The contents of the curiosity shop and second-hand store at the base of the rocket are equally fascinating.

►Continue down 35th and turn right onto Fremont Avenue North. This area features a succession of antique and vintage-clothing stores and ethnic restaurants. Ahead is the Fremont Bridge. According to some disgruntled residents, the drawbridge opens for everything including rowboats— or, if there are no rowboats, whenever more than four cars are approaching the bridge from either side.

►Before you reach the bridge, turn left onto North 34th Street and cross Fremont Avenue North to Costa's Opa. While passing the popular restaurant, look across the street to your right at the sculpture Waiting for the Interurban. On your left as you continue down North 34th is PCC Natural Market, a co-op that is open to the general public.

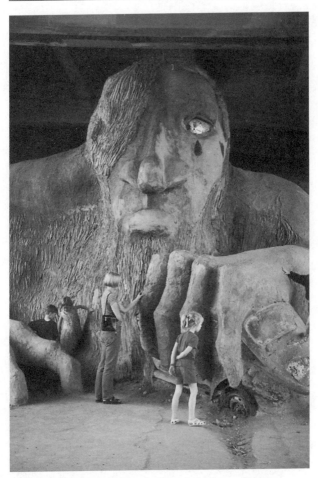

*The two-ton Fremont Troll lurks beneath the Aurora Bridge.*

## Funky Fremont

The Rocket: When members of the Fremont business community learned that they occupied the center of the universe, they decided they needed a unique landmark to celebrate the fact. They found one in an Army surplus store in Seattle—a Korean-built, 53-foot rocket that had served as a front-door display. The rocket was rescued, repaired, and improved by John Hoge.

According to the community's "hysterical marker," at 9 A.M. on June 3, 1994, "the rocket made a perfect five-minute sub-orbital flight from the Fremont Rocket Works to the center of the universe" at North 35th Street and Evanston Avenue North. When the rocket is in launch mode, neon laser pods flash on the fins and steam vapor pours out of the rocket base.

The Troll: In 1989, the Fremont Arts Council sought some imaginative work of art to occupy a space underneath the Aurora Bridge, a spot that otherwise might become a public eyesore. Sculptor Steve Badanes's project was the overwhelming choice. The Fremont Troll was sculpted from two tons of reinforced concrete. The creature is the centerpiece of the community's "Trolloween" celebration.

Lenin's Statue: The 8-ton, 18-foot-tall bronze statue was created by Slovakian sculptor Emil Venkov, who took 10 years to complete it after receiving a commission from the Czechoslovakian Communist Party in 1978. It was discovered face down in a Slovakian city dump in 1993 by Lew Carpenter, a Seattle-area man teaching in Eastern Europe at the time.

It cost Carpenter almost $30,000 dollars to ship the statue to Seattle. He failed in efforts to sell it, and upon his death Fremont welcomed this new resident to a perch in front of the Taco del Mar eatery, at North 36th Street and Evanston Avenue North. Why? To prove that "art outlives politics," according to Fremont sculptor Peter Bevis, who supervised the project.

Waiting for the Interurban: This famous piece of public art is located at the north end of the Fremont Bridge. Sculptor Richard Beyer created the work in 1978. It depicts in stone some commuters of long ago waiting for the Interurban railway, which once ran past this spot. Whenever there is a celebration in Fremont, the commuters are crowned with party hats. When the cold winds blow, residents rush out to supply the statues with mufflers and knit caps. One of the commuters was created with a dog's face. Some longtime residents claim it represents a critic of Beyer's early work.

➤At the intersection of North 34th and Aurora Avenue North, it is almost obligatory that you turn left and walk two blocks up a steep grade to view the Fremont Troll, who is crouched underneath the Aurora Bridge. You can pass up this side trip, but if you do, you had better not remain in Fremont after dark, when the troll begins to roam.

➤Once you have exchanged pleasantries with the troll, return to the bottom of the hill and History House, which contains interesting photographs and historical data.

➤Turn left onto North 34th Street again and continue east toward Gasworks Park. On your left are some recently constructed apartment houses, which have tremendous views of Lake Union and downtown Seattle.

➤Cross Stone Way Avenue North and link up with a pedestrian path, which takes you back to Gasworks Park. When you complete the walk, you automatically become an honorary citizen of Fremont. Delibertas Quirkas!

*walk* 6

# Ballard

     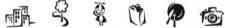

**General location**: About 4 miles northwest of downtown Seattle.

**Special attractions:** Views of yachts and working boats passing through locks between fresh water and Puget Sound; salmon and steelhead ladders and viewing rooms; Fisherman's Terminal; and downtown Ballard, Seattle's Scandinavian community.

**Difficulty rating:** Moderate; flat, but 1 mile of route is on the shoulder of city streets.

**Distance:** 4 miles.

**Estimated time:** 1.5 hours.

**Services:** Public restrooms at the locks and also at Fisherman's Terminal; restaurants at Fisherman's Terminal and in downtown Ballard.

# Ballard

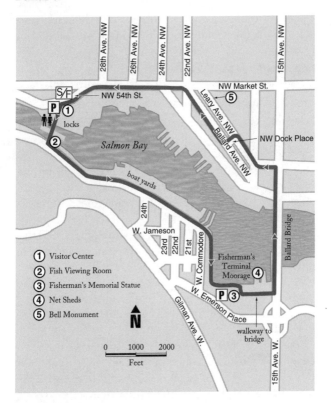

① Visitor Center
② Fish Viewing Room
③ Fisherman's Memorial Statue
④ Net Sheds
⑤ Bell Monument

**Restrictions:** Dogs must be leashed and their droppings picked up.

**For more information:** Contact the U.S. Army Corps of Engineers visitor center or the Ballard Chamber of Commerce.

**Getting started:** From the downtown waterfront, drive north on Elliott Avenue West, which becomes 15th Avenue West.

After crossing the Ballard Bridge, take the Ballard exit and continue straight ahead; then turn left onto Northwest Market Street. Veer left onto Northwest 54th Street. Turn left into the free parking lot at the Hiram M. Chittenden Locks.

**Public transportation:** Take Metro Transit Bus 17, which runs north on Fourth Avenue in downtown Seattle to 32nd Avenue Northwest and Northwest 54th Street.

**Overview:** The Lake Washington Ship Canal and Hiram M. Chittenden Locks dramatically transformed commerce and transportation in and around the Seattle area when they officially opened in 1917. And what an opening it was on July 4 of that year, highlighted by a parade of boats headed by the USS Roosevelt, flagship of Admiral Robert E. Peary's North Pole expedition.

The canal was built to link Lake Washington and Lake Union to Puget Sound. The locks lowered the water level in the freshwater lakes by as much as 20 feet. Before the water transportation corridor was created, trains carrying coal and lumber inched around the shores of Lake Washington, and boats in the Pacific fishing fleet had no freshwater moorage in this area.

Now, a 700-boat fishing fleet is headquartered at Fisherman's Terminal, within the canal. Cars, trucks, and trains can still pass over the canal on bridges that rise with the toot of a horn at the approach of sailboats or large working vessels.

On this walk, you will cross the locks, travel through Fisherman's Terminal, and then glimpse the best view of the canal from the top of the Ballard Bridge. The walk connects back to the locks via downtown Ballard, once an independent community that lured a great many immigrants from Scandinavia. Along the way, you may spot ocean-going vessels with names like Torddenskjold and Courageous, a yacht named C'Toy, or fishing boats named Tuition and Miss Conception. You might even glimpse the Never Again II.

The part of the canal that draws hundreds of thousands of visitors each year includes two navigation locks, a fish ladder, a botanical garden, a visitor center and bookstore, and a spillway dam. Sixty employees of the U.S. Army Corps of Engineers regulate boat traffic. The locks are open 24 hours a day, seven days a week. In an average year, 80,000 boats, barges, and log rafts pass between salt and fresh water.

The 21-step fish ladder allows sockeye, chinook, and coho salmon, plus cutthroat trout and steelhead, to return to spawning areas around Lake Washington. The fish struggling up the ladder can be viewed through six lighted windows below water level.

For a time it appeared that the $2.1 million ladder project would become an extremely expensive seafood cafe for sea

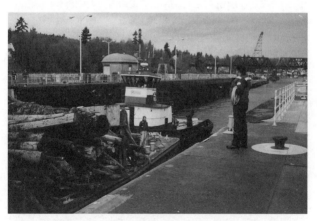

*A tugboat tows a timber barge through the Hiram M. Chittenden Locks at Ballard.*

lions. The pinnipeds would congregate just below the spill-way and would frequently rise out of the waters with struggling salmon locked in their jaws. The most eager eater was dubbed Herschel the Sea Lion. He and his friends were captured and shipped to California, only to return. Attempts have been made to scare them off with underwater explosions and with the introduction of a fiberglass orca, or killer whale, which resembled a giant bathtub toy. It was dubbed Fake Willy. When it, too, proved unsuccessful, it was removed.

## the walk

➤From the parking area, walk through the main entrance to the Chittenden Locks and into a parklike setting. You may want to spend some time at the visitor center, which will be on your left about 100 feet from the entrance. It is open daily during the summer and Thursdays through Mondays the remainder of the year. If it is closed, you can pick up literature about the locks in the administration building, farther down the walkway.

You will also want to spend some time at the locks watching the shuttling boats, from kayaks to barges piled 50 feet high with crab pots and headed for Alaska.

➤Cross the locks on the narrow bridges and be on the lookout for sea lions, which like to feed on the salmon and steelhead. The final bridge spans a spillway. Beyond it are fish viewing rooms, where you can get an underwater look at the fish ladders.

➤From the fish viewing rooms, continue on to the top of the ramp and then turn left onto West Commodore Way. The sidewalk passes a row of apartment complexes with views of the locks.

As you enter the industrial area, you must walk on the left side of the road, facing traffic, for half a mile. To your left, you will see adventure cruise ships, crab boats, tugs, and ancient freighters being refitted, repainted, and rebuilt. A small sign marks the entrance to Fisherman's Terminal.

►Turn right immediately after entering the moorage area and head toward the large Fisherman's Terminal sign on top of the tallest building. Here, you can venture out onto the various finger piers to sightsee, take pictures, or chat with a sailor mending a net or tinkering with a greasy engine. On second thought, better not interrupt the guy immersed to his elbows in grease.

Signs at dockside will help you identify the different vessels and gear and all the varieties of fish caught by the Seattle fleet.

The terminal has been home to the Seattle fishing fleet since 1913, and it provides year-round moorage to more than 700 commercial vessels ranging from 30 to 300 feet long. The fleet includes gill netters, trollers, purse seiners, halibut long liners, crab boats, trawlers, and fish processors. Because the terminal is located in fresh water, the vessels are not subject to tides and other problems related to saltwater, like corrosion and wood-eating worms. Because of the mild climate, fishermen can make repairs year-round.

Looming above the docks is the Seattle Fisherman's Memorial, a statue of a fisherman pulling in a catch. It is dedicated to members of the local fishing fleet lost at sea and to their surviving relatives. The sculpture is the work of Ronald Petty, and he served as his own model for the work, partly because no working fisherman wanted to cast himself in the role of the lost seaman. On the column below the figure, Petty depicted 32 different forms of sea life. He said he spent countless hours doing research since he knew his work would be judged by a critical, if unofficial, jury.

➤Exit Fisherman's Terminal by the main entrance at the big Chinook's sign and turn left onto West Commodore Way. The walkway takes you past some big net sheds and onto Ballard Bridge.

➤Cross the bridge on the left side, looking down at the fishing fleet, and, at the far side, keep walking until you reach Leary Avenue Northwest.

➤Do not cross the street. Turn left onto Leary. The street will eventually angle to the right.

➤Turn left onto Northwest Dock Place.

➤After one block, turn right onto Ballard Avenue Northwest at Bad Albert's Tavern. You will pass several colorful taverns in the next couple of blocks, including some featuring live jazz or Irish music.

➤Pass to the right of a large monument that commemorates the annexation of Ballard by Seattle. On your right is

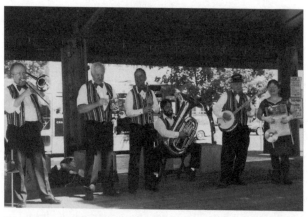

*The community of Ballard celebrates its Scandinavian heritage in many colorful ways.*

**A Working Town, You Betcha**

In Ballard, you can buy a Danish flag, a block of geitost cheese, a Norwegian bunad costume, two pounds of lute-fisk, or a bumper sticker that reads, "You Can Always Tell a Swede, But You Can't Tell Him Much."

Residents of this colorful community seem to treasure their heritage, even the gentle insults. Many of their distant and not-so-distant relatives arrived on Salmon Bay in the late 1800s, attracted by jobs with the fishing fleet or in shingle mills, where Ballard's output led the world. After the Great Fire of 1889, Ballard mills worked overtime, providing logs, boards, and shingles needed to rebuild downtown Seattle. At one time, 30 sawmills operated around the clock.

Ballard was known as a working man's town, with a lot of rough edges. But it was not as rough as the life many of the pioneers left behind in the small towns of Scandinavia. Some of them originally settled east of the Mississippi and then relocated in Ballard after the eastern forests were depleted.

The reputation as a working stiff's town is less deserved in Ballard today. In 1907, the community boasted 23 bars and 22 churches. Now the growth industry is coffee bars. Office workers and executives from central Seattle have discovered in Ballard a picturesque community with friendly neighborhoods and a short commute to their office buildings.

In the early 1900s, Ballard was still an independent city, but on May 30, 1907, the community was annexed by Seattle. The bell in town hall chimed the news, and it reportedly sounded like a funeral toll. You can still find the bell at the corner of Ballard Avenue Northwest and 22nd Avenue Northwest. That is where the town hall once stood. It is now the location of a historical monument dedicated in 1976 by Sweden's King Karl Gustaf XVI and the mayor of Seattle, creating the Ballard Avenue Historic District.

Jones Brothers Meat Market, another long-standing institution. Beyond Jones Brothers is a large Scandinavian mural in a small courtyard, which serves as a bus shelter and as a stage during local celebrations.

➤You can head to your right up Northwest Market if you wish to explore some of the Scandinavian souvenir shops, but our route goes left on Market and back to the locks. Across Market, as you head toward the locks, is Olsen's Scandinavian Foods, where you can load up on lutefisk. Eventually you will pass an inflatable-boat company on your left.

➤Bear left on Northwest 54th to the locks. At the end of the walk, you will encounter the Lock Spot Café and Tavern and the Stone Gardens indoor rock-climbing facility. If you still feel the need to work off a few calories, you can hang by your teeth from a piton. Or you can go the opposite route: buy some fish and chips from Lock Spot and take them to a bench in the botanical garden, which adjoins the ship canal, or to a bench along the locks.

*walk* **7**

# West Seattle

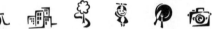

**General location:** Across Elliott Bay from the city center via West Seattle Bridge.

**Special attractions:** Nautical views, beaches, several restaurants.

**Difficulty rating:** Moderate; flat, paved sidewalks and asphalt pedestrian lanes.

**Distance:** 5.7 miles.

**Estimated time:** 2.5 hours.

**Services:** Several restaurants, restrooms, and drinking fountains at Seacrest Marina Park and on Alki Beach.

**Restrictions:** Leash and scoop laws for pets enforced. No pets on swimming beaches.

**For more information:** Contact the Seattle Parks Department, Alki Point Light Station, or the West Seattle Historical Society.

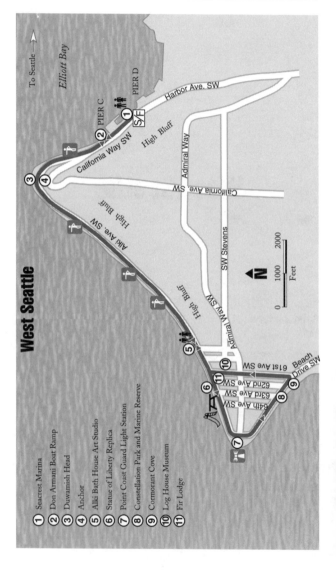

**West Seattle**

To Seattle →

Elliott Bay

PIER D

PIER C

S/F

Harbor Ave. SW

California Way SW

High Bluff

Admiral Way

California Ave. SW

SW Stevens

High Bluff

Admiral Way SW

High Bluff

Alki Ave. SW

61st Ave SW

62nd Ave SW

63rd Ave SW

64th Ave SW

Beach Drive SW

N

0      1000      2000
Feet

① Seacrest Marina
② Don Armani Boat Ramp
③ Duwamish Head
④ Anchor
⑤ Alki Bath House Art Studio
⑥ Statue of Liberty Replica
⑦ Point Coast Guard Light Station
⑧ Constellation Park and Marine Reserve
⑨ Cormorant Cove
⑩ Log House Museum
⑪ Fir Lodge

**Getting started:** From Interstate 5 Southbound, exit onto West Seattle Bridge. Continue over the main span and move into the right lane. Take the Harbor Avenue Southwest exit ramp. (Do not confuse Harbor Avenue with Harbor Island. Both exit off the West Seattle Bridge.) Follow Harbor Avenue Southwest past Salty's on Alki Restaurant to Seacrest Marina Park. There is free parking with a two-hour limit in the marina lot. There is often curbside parking available on Harbor Avenue with no time limit.

**Public transportation:** Board southbound Metro Transit Bus 37 on Second Avenue, in downtown Seattle. Get off at Seacrest Marina Park on Harbor Avenue Southwest.

**Overview:** If the sun is shining, the view across Elliott Bay from West Seattle is breathtaking. But the sun made infrequent appearances in the winter of 1851-1852, when the members of the Denny party homesteaded in tents on what is now Alki Beach. The men and women in that pioneer party expected to find a completed cabin, and they anticipated a warm and enthusiastic welcome from David Denny, who had preceded them as part of a two-man advance party.

Instead, what the pioneers from the schooner *Exact* found when they landed during a driving rain was an unroofed cabin and a one-man plague in the person of David Denny. He was suffering from neuralgia, malaria, and an axe wound to his foot. He was also hungry. Skunks had raided his provisions.

The pioneers almost immediately realized that the beach was too shallow to accommodate large ships. They hoped to make their fortune by cutting and selling the trees that covered the land, so it was essential that they find a deepwater port to accommodate the ocean freighters they hoped to lure to this section of Puget Sound.

In February 1852, David Denny's older brother Arthur, along with John Bell and Carson Boren, paddled around the bay in a small boat. They took soundings using a clothesline with a bundle of horseshoes attached to one end. The site they finally selected for a new city is not difficult to identify today, because, across the bay, Seattle skyscrapers rise like towers in the Land of Oz. In fact, Emerald City is now the unofficial nickname used by civic boosters.

On this walk along the shoreline of West Seattle—around the Duwamish Head and down the beach to Alki Point—it is possible to revisit the past and get a glimpse of the Denny party's dream. The pioneers originally named their settlement New York. More than 50 years later, after Seattle had been settled and renamed, an amusement park was built at Duwamish Head. It was given the same name as an attraction then operating at Coney Island, New York: Luna Park. By 1914, New York's Luna Park had burned down, and its namesake in West Seattle had closed.

Imaginative exhibits and viewfinders erected along this route recall images of the Denny party's rowboat, the White City Carnival Joy Wheel at Luna Park, and a tent camp that sprouted on the beach after the Klondike gold rush.

West Seattle was incorporated in 1902, when passenger ferries and an electric railroad carried visitors and commuters to and from Seattle. Only five years later, it was annexed by Seattle. Today, commuters cross the Duwamish River via soaring bridges. Even when the sun is not shining, the view is pretty impressive.

## the walk

►Start at Seacrest Marina Park, which has a restaurant, sea-kayak rentals, accessible restrooms, and a fishing dock. With

Elliott Bay on your right, walk along Harbor Avenue Southwest. You have a choice of the curbside sidewalk or another walkway along the seawall.

Pause at one of the viewpoints overlooking Elliott Bay. Straight ahead is downtown Seattle. The flash of orange to your right marks the container terminals beside the dry docks of Harbor Island. To the right of the Seattle skyscrapers are twin stadiums for the city's professional baseball and football teams. To the left of the skyscrapers, notice the Space Needle and the giant grain terminals fronting Queen Anne Hill. Farther to the left is the bridge that leads to Magnolia Bluff.

➤Just past the Don Armani Boat Ramp on your right, the seawall and curbside sidewalks merge. You are now entering an area known as the Duwamish Head. Passenger ferryboats once darted back and forth across Elliott Bay, shuttling families between Seattle and Luna Park. The first of a series of interpretive signs posted along the sidewalk recites the history of the 12-acre amusement park that opened here in 1907. It was built on pilings that are still visible at low tide. What appear to be high-powered field glasses at the historical markers are actually viewers that superimpose scenes from yesteryear over the actual contemporary landscape.

The Ferris wheel at Luna Park is featured on one of the two viewers located at this first site. The other shows a bundle of horseshoes attached to a clothesline. This was the "depth finder" favored by members of the Denny party when they surveyed Elliott Bay.

➤Follow Harbor Avenue Southwest as it curves left around the point of Duwamish Head and becomes Alki Avenue Southwest. At this transition point, there is a large anchor from an unidentified sailing vessel that was recovered from

**of interest**

### Elliott Bay

The body of water now identified as Elliott Bay was explored by Captain George Vancouver in 1792 and was named for Midshipman Sam Elliott, a member of the 1841 Wilkes Expedition. Elliott was the first person to chart the bay, and he reported that it was 100 fathoms, or about 600 feet, deep. He recommended it as a safe anchorage.

Twice daily, Elliott Bay is flushed by the tides with vast amounts of cold water. Thus, even in the shallows in midsummer, the temperature fails to top 50 degrees.

Harbor seals are frequently spotted in Elliott Bay. Orcas are seen less often. Also living in these waters are 75 species of fish, several rare types of crabs, and the largest octopuses in the world. They measure up to 16 feet long and weigh up to 600 pounds.

Early visitors to Elliott Bay included the *Beaver*, which was the flagship of the Hudson's Bay Company fleet and the first steamer on the West Coast. Paddle wheelers like the *Eliza Anderson* also occasionally entered the bay. Clipper ships and lumber schooners soon arrived to fulfill the original dreams of the pioneers in the Denny party.

Ferryboats once raced on Elliott Bay, a tradition that has been revived and is now a feature of Maritime Week in May.

these waters by the Northwest Divers Club. A plaque points out that, on the evening of November 18, 1906, 2 miles due west of this site, the steamer *Dix* collided with an Alaskan steamer while traveling from Seattle to Port Blakely. The accident claimed 42 lives.

If you visit this waterfront at noon, you are liable to see sailboats, ocean freighters, ferryboats, hydrofoils, working

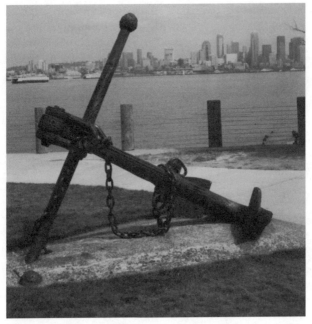

*The Seattle skyline and Elliott Bay are the backdrop for this anchor, which once belonged to a 19th-century schooner.*

tugboats, Coast Guard cutters, and the *Princess Marguerite* ferrying people to Seattle from Victoria, British Columbia.

➤Continue to follow Alki Avenue Southwest. The area on your left graphically shows the transition under way along this thoroughfare. A few beach cabins still remain, but luxury condominiums have replaced many of them.

➤Bear right as you enter a mile-long stretch where bicyclists, wheelchair users, and skaters are separated by pavement markers from walkers and joggers. Just remember when heading this direction, "heels" stay right and "wheels" keep left.

The history and revival of canoe racing by Northwest Native Americans is featured on the next interpretive sign. The traditional racing canoe had 11 rowers capable of taking 60 strokes per minute. The viewer at this site focuses on the waters off Alki Beach, with the image of a racing canoe superimposed.

Extensive beds of eelgrass lie off Alki Beach and are mentioned on yet another interpretive sign along this route. Only sugar cane converts sunshine into more living substance than does eelgrass, which provides food and habitat for 200 species of marine animals, 75 species of fish, and more than 200 species of birds.

Another viewpoint focuses upon the contributions of Japanese Americans to the community of West Seattle and recalls the tragic days during World War II when residents of Japanese heritage were forced to relocate to internment camps.

The beach to your right widens at an area where volleyball tournaments are held during the spring and summer. "Restaurant row" begins at about this point, on the opposite side of Alki Avenue Southwest.

Originally a bathhouse, the structure across the street from Spud Fish and Chips now serves as a public art studio. "Art for Sale" signs are frequently posted by the painters and sculptors who work inside. There are also public restrooms and drinking fountains at the Alki Bath House Art Studio.

A broad strip of grass between the sidewalk and the beach begins just beyond the bathhouse. It features picnic tables, stone stairways down to the sand, and more historical markers regarding the beach and the adjoining waters. A small-scale replica of the Statue of Liberty occupies a place of prominence in this picnic area. The Boy Scouts presented the replica to the city on February 23, 1952.

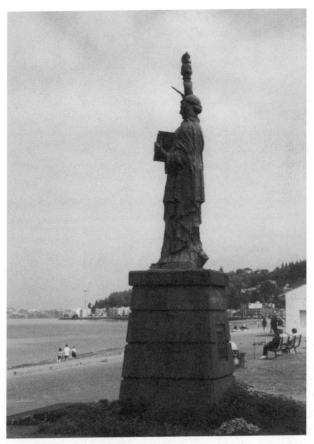

*A small-scale replica of the Statue of Liberty marks the spot where the founders of Seattle first stepped ashore in 1851.*

Just beyond this landmark, note the stone pylon identifying the birthplace of Seattle. "At this place on 18 November, 1851, there landed from the schooner *Exact*, the little colony which developed into the city of Seattle," reads the dedication. The names of the original settlers follow.

➤After you leave the picnic grounds, cross Alki Avenue Southwest to the sidewalk on the opposite side. To avoid this and other potentially hazardous street crossings, wheelchair users are advised to turn back at this point and return via Alki Avenue Southwest to the starting and finishing point at Seacrest Marina Park.

➤Follow the sidewalk on the left side of Alki Avenue Southwest through the left turn where Alki becomes Beach Drive Southwest.

➤Cross the street once again at the sign pointing to the Alki Point Coast Guard Light Station. The lighthouse and support buildings are open to the public for tours from noon to 4 P.M. on Saturdays, Sundays, and most holidays from May through September.

➤Follow the sidewalk on the right side of the street as you continue along Beach Drive. To your right, in Puget Sound, you can see Blake Island and larger Vashon Island to its left. Benches face the sound. The beach here is rocky, but the tide pools are worth exploring when the tide is low. There are stairways that lead from the sidewalk to the beach. On the left, across the street, is a municipal water-treatment facility.

➤The intersection of Beach Drive and 63rd Avenue Southwest marks the entrance to Constellation Park and Marine Reserve. This educational resource offers displays linking marine biology and environmental conservation "within the context of art, mythology, and astronomy." A highlight is the Avenue of Stars, which features bronze stars, set into the sidewalk, depicting the 27 constellations that are visible from the park at night.

➤Continue up Beach Drive to 61st Avenue Southwest, site of the neighborhood park known as Cormorant Cove, which offers beach access.

➤At this point, cross the street and walk away from the beach on 61st Avenue Southwest. There is a stop sign where 61st crosses busy Admiral Way. Wait for a break in the traffic before continuing on 61st to its intersection with Southwest Stevens Street.

Note the signs on your left identifying the Log House Museum, which features memorabilia from and photographs of West Seattle's pioneer days. This was the location of the stables for Fir Lodge, which is farther down 61st Avenue Southwest. A gift shop is located behind the museum.

➤Continue to Fir Lodge at 2717 61st Avenue Southwest. This structure was built in 1903 of logs salvaged from Alki Beach. It is now occupied by the Alki Homestead Restaurant, once praised by *USA Today* for the excellence of its pan-fried chicken.

➤At the intersection of 61st and Alki Avenue Southwest, turn right onto Alki and return along the beach back to Seacrest Marina Park. The return walk offers fresh views across busy Elliott Bay with downtown Seattle as a backdrop.

*walk* 8

# Volunteer Park and the Broadway District

**General location:** About 5 miles northeast of the city center.

**Special attractions:** Interesting architecture, art museum, conservatory, observation tower, several restaurants and shops, children's playground and wading pool in Volunteer Park.

**Difficulty rating:** Easy; flat, paved sidewalks except for a short distance on park paths.

**Distance:** 2.5 miles.

**Estimated time:** 1.5 hours.

**Services:** Several restaurants and fast-food stands, restrooms in park.

**Restrictions:** Leash and scoop laws for pets enforced.

# Volunteer Park and the Broadway District

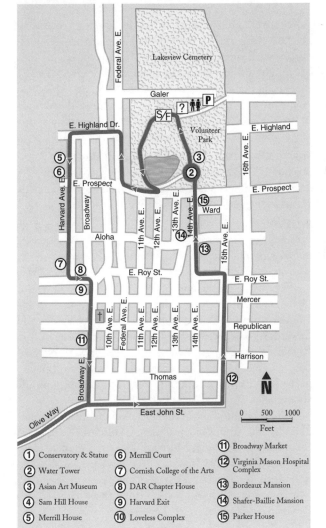

① Conservatory & Statue
② Water Tower
③ Asian Art Museum
④ Sam Hill House
⑤ Merrill House
⑥ Merrill Court
⑦ Cornish College of the Arts
⑧ DAR Chapter House
⑨ Harvard Exit
⑩ Loveless Complex
⑪ Broadway Market
⑫ Virginia Mason Hospital Complex
⑬ Bordeaux Mansion
⑭ Shafer-Baillie Mansion
⑮ Parker House

**For more information:** Contact the Seattle Asian Art Museum or the Seattle Parks Department.

**Getting started:** From downtown Seattle, head north on Fourth Avenue. Turn right onto Olive Way and then left onto Broadway. Bear right at Roy Street onto 10th Avenue East. Turn right at Prospect Street East, which leads to the Volunteer Park entrance. Drive into the park, pass the Asian Art Museum, and park near the statue of William H. Seward. There is no parking lot, but curbside parking is usually available on the main road through Volunteer Park.

**Public transportation:** Board Metro Transit Bus 10 at Fourth Avenue and Pike Street in downtown Seattle. Get off at 15th Avenue East and East Galer Street. Follow the pathway into the park to the Seward statue.

**Overview:** This walk begins around 1850, passes quickly through the 20th century, and then returns to about 1900 and Volunteer Park, which was named in honor of veterans who had volunteered to serve in the Spanish-American War.

The glimpse of the mid-1800s is afforded by the Volunteer Park Conservatory, which was designed to resemble London's Crystal Palace, and by the statue of William H. Seward, who negotiated the 1867 purchase of Alaska from Russia. The walk passes out of Volunteer Park, through sedate neighborhoods of historic homes, and onto glitzy, fast-paced Broadway, one of the city centers for dining, nightlife, shopping, and people watching.

In addition to the conservatory, which houses cactuses, orchids, and various tropical plants, Volunteer Park is also the site of the Asian Art Museum. This protomodern structure was built in 1932 to house the city's principal collection of paintings and sculptures. When a second Seattle Art Museum opened downtown in 1991, the Volunteer Park facility began to focus on Asian art.

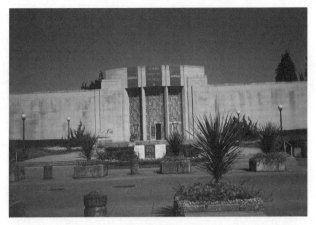

*The Asian Art Museum, built in 1932, was originally intended to showcase a wide variety of paintings and sculptures that belonged to the City of Seattle.*

Opposite the entrance to the Asian Art Museum is a 9-foot-tall granite sculpture, the Black Sun, created by Isamu Noguchi in 1968. It may not have been the artist's intention to provide an enormous granite "frame" for the Space Needle, but that Seattle landmark is in the center of the circle created by the sculpture when you glimpse it from the museum steps.

There are dahlia gardens next to the conservatory. Behind the gardens are a children's playground and restrooms.

The master plan for Volunteer Park was presented to the city council in 1887 and was opposed by Seattle's superintendent of parks, who thought the location too remote and difficult to maintain. But by the mid-1880s, a streetcar ran from central Seattle to the Broadway District, and many wealthy residents began to build estates on the surrounding lands. A bandstand for summer concerts once stood on the land now occupied by the Asian Art Museum.

# the walk

➤As you face the statue of William H. Seward and the conservatory behind it, begin the walk on the gravel path that leads off to the left and downhill through a heavily forested part of Volunteer Park.

➤Cross a feeder road just past two tennis courts. The path continues beside this unmarked park road, passes under two giant oak trees, and ends at a stop sign marking the park exit, at the intersection of 12th Avenue East and East Prospect Street.

➤Cross Prospect, turn right, and head downhill on this winding street lined with stately houses and towering trees.

➤Turn right off Prospect onto Federal Avenue East.

➤Walk one block and turn left onto East Highland Drive.

➤At busy 10th Avenue East, wait for a traffic break to cross. The castlelike structure at 814 East Highland Drive is the Sam Hill House, which once belonged to the nephew of railroad baron James J. Hill, who owned the Great Northern and Northern Pacific railroads. Although rundown and unimpressive today, this concrete re-creation of an 18th-century manor house has two stories below the street level, as well as two above. It was reputedly built so that Sam and Mary Hill could properly welcome Crown Prince Albert of Belgium. Unfortunately, the prince canceled his plans to visit Seattle.

Sam Hill later built a duplicate of Hill House on the Columbia River near the Washington-Oregon border. He named the country home Maryhill, after his wife.

From this point on East Highland Drive, you can glimpse St. Mark's Episcopal Cathedral, built in 1930.

➤At the end of East Highland, turn left onto Harvard Avenue East. The original residents of the prestigious neighborhood you are now entering were heavily involved in banking and railroads. Between 1905 and 1910, they financed the construction of Colonial, Tudor, and Georgian Revival mansions in what is now known as the Harvard-Belmont Historic District.

Of interest is the Merrill House, built in 1910 at 919 Harvard Avenue East. The address is placed above the entrance in Roman numerals. The Georgian Revival house was designed by prominent eastern architect Charles Platt. It included a formal garden and carriage house.

Next to the Merrill House, at 917 Harvard, is Merrill Court. This tasteful, three-story, brick townhouse surrounds a small park. The designers were awarded a city citation in 1991 for promoting "Housing Designs that Work."

➤The three former residences in the 700 block comprise Harvard House, now occupied by offices of the Cornish College of the Arts. The center of this small "campus" is the Spanish-style structure at the intersection of Harvard and East Roy Street. A former sheep farmer who moved to Seattle in 1900 helped his daughter to establish an arts institute in 1914 at Broadway and Pine in downtown Seattle. The daughter, Nellie Cornish, moved the college to this location in 1920. The school once included painter Mark Tobey and choreographer Martha Graham among its faculty and is still a leading center for arts education in Seattle.

➤Turn left off Harvard onto East Roy Street. At 800 East Roy is the Rainier Chapter House of the Daughters of the American Revolution. It resembles a southern mansion and is a popular site for weddings and other social soirees.

Directly across the street from the DAR site is the Harvard Exit Theater, formerly the Women's Century Club.

Theater patrons often arrive early to read or relax in the former drawing room or to indulge in a quiet game of chess, interrupted only by the sounds and smells drifting in from the popcorn machine in the lobby.

Next to the Rainier Chapter House, starting on East Roy Street and winding around the corner onto Broadway, is the Loveless complex of shops and apartments. Although built during the Great Depression, the cinder- and concrete-block complex resembles a cluster of English cottages complete with round stair towers and balconies that overlook a courtyard accessible from Broadway.

➤Cross East Roy Street and head down Broadway. On the opposite side of Roy, you will pass the Deluxe, which has long been a popular, low-priced steak and hamburger emporium. Just past the Deluxe, look for bronze "footprints" in the sidewalk. There are eight such examples of Jack Mackie's public art along Broadway. Each is a graphic illustration of a different dance step, complete with numbers and arrows. This first one shows you how to dance "The Lindy."

➤There are a couple of dozen restaurants in the next three or four blocks of Broadway, along with specialty shops and three giant supermarkets. On the corner of Broadway and Republican Street is Plymouth Congregational Church. Diagonally across from the church is the entrance to the block-long Broadway Market. Your first sniff as you enter suggests incense from an international bazaar, the scent of a florist's blooms, espresso brewing, raw leather from a shoe-repair shop, fragrances from a perfumery, and tantalizing odors from food stands. There is a newsstand, a multiplex theater, record shops, a candy shop, clothing stores, a Fred Meyer outlet, and lots of underground parking. You leave the market through an exit at mid-block.

➤Continue on Broadway to Olive Way.

➤Turn left onto Olive Way and cross Broadway. Olive Way then becomes East John Street. At the end of the street, off 15th Avenue East, looms the mammoth Virginia Mason-Group Health Cooperative hospital and clinic complex.

The brick apartment building and courtyard at 1405 East John Street were the work of developer Fred Anhalt, who was well known in this part of Seattle in the 1930s for projects conceived in the Olde English style.

➤Turn left onto 15th Avenue East and head past the relatively new Safeway superstore. Just past the hospital and clinic complex, you will enter yet another "restaurant row."

The building at 15th and Harrison, which once housed Fire Station 7, now serves as a video outlet. "Challenge Authority" seems to be the unofficial motto of the Red and Black Book Collective, which has operated for more than 25 years at 432 15th Avenue East.

➤Turn left off 15th onto East Roy Street.

➤Walk 1 block and turn right onto 14th Avenue East. You are now entering what was once known as Millionaires' Row, one of the first "gated communities" in the West. The gate at 14th and Roy is long gone, but an atmosphere of quiet grace still prevails, especially at the former Thomas Bordeaux residence at 806 14th Avenue East. Bordeaux made his fortune in lumber and banking. His half-timbered Tyrolian mansion with its decorative tower, built in 1903, is now almost hidden behind holly bushes, vines, and red maple trees that line the boulevard.

A plaque identifies the Shafer-Baillie Mansion, 907 14th Avenue East, as a bed-and-breakfast inn. Austrian-born Julius Shafer arrived in this country at the age of 12. He and his brother eventually settled in Seattle and opened a secondhand clothing store with $700 in savings. When news of the Klondike gold strike reached the city, the Shafer brothers shifted their emphasis to outfitting prospectors headed north by ship from Seattle. With his profits, Julius not only built this mansion, which has 13 rooms and 10 baths, but he also financed the construction of a 10-story office building downtown. Note the five-globed lighting fixtures that illuminate the mansion's entrance and garden.

One of the most prominent structures on Millionaires' Row, at 14th and East Prospect Street, is the stark white, Colonial-style Parker House. It was built in 1909 for $150,000. That investment bought owner George Parker a 30-room mansion with Corinthian columns, seven fireplaces, five covered porches, and an adjoining coach house. Some of Parker's other investments were less profitable. In 1910, he was sentenced to McNeil Island Federal Prison for stock fraud.

Millionaires' Row ends at the Parker House and the entrance to Volunteer Park.

➤Enter the park and walk toward the water tower on the path that curves right around this looming structure. Two signs lead you toward the "Water Tower, Observation Deck and Olmsted Exhibit."

➤A steep path leads uphill to the tower, which can hold almost 900,000 gallons of water. Its observation deck is open daily from 10 A.M. until dusk. Be forewarned: There are 106 steps leading up the curved staircase to the observation deck, but the climb is rewarding. Windows built into the top level of the tower look out on the skyscrapers of downtown Seattle, the Space Needle, ships in Elliott Bay, the Evergreen Point Floating Bridge across Lake Washington, and the eastside communities of Bellevue and Kirkland.

An exhibit on the same level highlights the career of Frederick Law Olmsted, Sr., described as "the father of landscape architecture." His work extended from the lawns of

## The Olmsted Master Plan

The Olmsted Brothers firm of New York City, which designed world-famous Central Park, was commissioned in 1903 to create a master plan for the Seattle park system.

Frederick Law Olmsted, Sr., the firm's founder, dispatched his stepson John to Seattle to fulfill the commission. John traveled throughout the city by carriage and streetcar and on foot. He climbed the major hills and inspected the city by boat before drafting a plan that called for 50 miles of boulevards and more than 2,000 acres of parkland. The plan led to the creation of a greenbelt that stretches across the city.

This greenbelt extends from Volunteer Park on one end through the University of Washington campus, Washington Park Arboretum, Ravenna Boulevard, Green Lake Park, and Woodland Park, across the ship canal to Discovery Park, and south along Magnolia Boulevard. From Magnolia Bluff, you can look across Elliott Bay to West Seattle, site of Schmitz Park Preserve, another piece of the Olmsted master plan.

Visit all of these parks, travel the tree-lined boulevards, and you will have glimpsed some, but not nearly all, of the influences the Olmsted Brothers exerted on Seattle.

The Olmsted design for Volunteer Park included formal gardens, circular drives, lily ponds, a central concourse, a music pavilion, and a conservatory, all adjacent to and complementing a city reservoir.

A room at the top of the park's brick-and-ivy covered water tower is devoted to an exhibit of drawings, photos, and charts connected with the Olmsted plan for Seattle parks.

Central Park in New York City to the parks and boulevards of Seattle.

➤Continue along the pathway that leads from the water tower into the park. The sidewalk through the central portion of the park passes between a reservoir and the old Seattle Art Museum, now dedicated to exhibits of Asian art.

➤Walk straight ahead past the museum, and you will be back at the conservatory and Seward statue, the starting and finishing point of this walk.

History buffs might want to visit Lakeview Cemetery, just north of Volunteer Park. Interred there is Princess Angeline, daughter of Chief Sealth, as well as members of many of Seattle's founding families, including Dennys, Mercers, Yeslers, Hortons, and Maynards. Also buried there are Bruce and Brandon Lee, the father and son film stars who both died at the height of their popularity.

*walk* 9

# Madison Park

  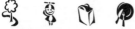 

**General location:** On the west shore of Lake Washington, about 6 miles northwest of the city center.

**Special attractions:** Estates, gardens, restaurants, upscale shops.

**Difficulty rating:** Moderate; some steep hills and unpaved paths.

**Distance:** 4.7 miles.

**Estimated time:** 2.5 hours.

**Services:** Restaurants and restrooms at Madison Park, restrooms at Madrona Park.

**Restrictions:** Leash and scoop laws for pets enforced.

**For more information:** Contact the Seattle Parks Department or the Madison Park Community Council.

**Getting started:** From downtown Seattle, head north on Interstate 5 and take the Washington Highway 520 (Bellevue)

# Madison Park

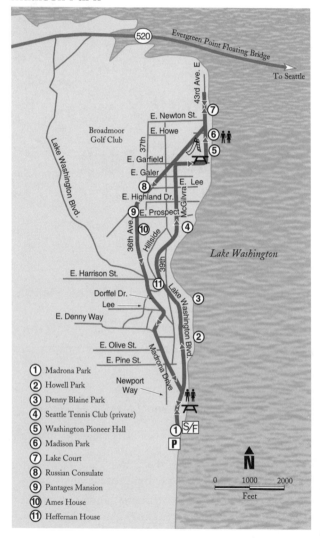

① Madrona Park
② Howell Park
③ Denny Blaine Park
④ Seattle Tennis Club (private)
⑤ Washington Pioneer Hall
⑥ Madison Park
⑦ Lake Court
⑧ Russian Consulate
⑨ Pantages Mansion
⑩ Ames House
⑪ Heffernan House

exit. After a quarter-mile, take the Montlake Boulevard exit, also marked "University of Washington." Stay in the right lane. Go straight through the traffic light after passing a sign for the Washington Park Arboretum. You are now on Lake Washington Boulevard, which takes you right through the arboretum and passes over Madison Avenue.

Continue on Lake Washington Boulevard as it winds steeply downhill and through a residential district to the shores of Lake Washington. You will come to a sign that reads "Madrona Park." Continue another 200 yards on Lake Washington Boulevard to a large lot where you may park for free. The parking area overlooks swim platforms and, in the distance, Mount Rainier.

**Public transportation:** From the city center, take Metro Transit Bus 2 south via Third Avenue to the end of the line. You can begin your walk at the end of the line (the Madrona bus turnaround) or walk south 300 yards along the Lake Washington shore to reach Madrona Park.

**Overview:** Near the west shore of Lake Washington, Seattle resembles a giant wedding cake, rising tier upon tier—or, more accurately, hill upon hill. From a boat anchored offshore, it might look as though builders had piled house upon house. Somehow these dwellings all manage to cling to these treasured sites with a view.

This walk past many of the grandest homes in the city proceeds up each topographical level, from the lakeside mansions on McGilvra Boulevard, uphill through posh Madison Park, where even the supermarket is carpeted, to turn-of-the-20th-century mansions erected in Washington Park by wealthy pioneers.

The route passes the Seattle Tennis Club, where the wait for a membership opening sometimes can last several years, and the Broadmoor Golf and Country Club, where memberships cost upwards of $100,000. The walk also offers a glimpse of exclusive Bush School, a private, preparatory school.

This tour provides compelling evidence that Judge John McGilvra, who practiced law with Abraham Lincoln in Chicago, made a wise choice when he left the courts and politics to become a real estate developer in Seattle. McGilvra donated 21 acres for the development of a lakeside park to adjoin the lots he was trying to sell. An amusement park— complete with pavilion, boathouse, and racetrack—was created at the end of a new streetcar line. This is where the community of Madison Park now stands. Until World War II, the area featured rows of "beach shacks" on small lots. Many of the lots are still small in Madison Park, but the price tags on the cottages that replaced the shacks are among the highest on the Seattle real estate market.

There is a "Gold Coast" along Lake Washington, beneath several layers of wedding-cake frosting.

# the walk

➤From Madrona Park, begin walking toward the brick bathhouse, which now houses a dance studio. Your route will alternate between sidewalk and dirt pathway.

➤After you pass the bathhouse, look to your left at the four-level residence dominated by picture windows. Note the house farther up the embankment, which has good views from two levels. This is typical of the way architects have maximized the views along this section of the lakefront.

To your right, across the lake, you can see the skyscrapers of downtown Bellevue. One hundred yards past the bathhouse, there are public restrooms and picnic tables. During daylight hours in the summer, food concessions operate in this part of Madrona Park.

➤Continue on a lakeshore path past a bus-turnaround circle marking the end of Madrona Avenue. Note the cluster of small homes across Lake Washington Boulevard to the left. They replaced similarly sized beach cottages that stood here when streetcars were the preferred method of transportation to the lakeshore.

➤When the dirt path ends, continue walking for a short distance on the marked bicycle-pedestrian route on the lake side of the boulevard. The sidewalk soon resumes and enters an area of expensive homes and manicured lawns along Lake Washington Boulevard.

Note the sign on your right indicating a pathway to lakeshore access at Howell Park. To the left, across the boulevard, a grassy area features park benches for the use of local residents or passing pedestrians.

➤At 168 Lake Washington Boulevard, you will see the entrance to a lakeside mansion flanked by tall palm trees. Note tiny Denny Blaine Park to your right. Grassy expanses in the park are illuminated on summer nights by globe streetlights. There is also parking and a path to the lakeshore here.

➤Cross Lake Washington Boulevard to the sidewalk on the other side. A mansion on the left is fronted by a formal rose garden.

➤Cross Lake Washington Boulevard again at a four-way stop and head up McGilvra Boulevard East. 39th Avenue East leads downhill to the lakeshore past another row of imposing residences. Eventually, 39th merges back into McGilvra.

Each mansion along McGilvra Boulevard East seems larger and grander than the last. Note the formal European-style garden and patio adjoining the residence at 430 McGilvra. View-obstructing walls and fences become less common as you continue up McGilvra, and the contrasting architectural styles, as well as lawns manicured like putting greens, give this area a charming, almost picture-book quality.

The towering tree in front of the residence at 700 McGilvra is a yellow poplar, or tulip tree. This hardwood, native to the eastern United States, was introduced to Washington by a few early pioneers. Often the trees were felled and hollowed out to create giant canoes for lake or river travel.

The social center of the McGilvra and Madison neighborhoods is the Seattle Tennis Club, on your right where the boulevard curves toward the lake. The private club features outdoor and indoor courts, a swimming pool, a beach, a dining hall, a ballroom, and offices.

➤Turn right off McGilvra Boulevard East onto East Garfield Street.

➤Turn left onto 43rd Avenue East. The high-rise Washington Park Tower and the smaller Park Shore next door were controversial projects when they were built. They preceded current zoning laws that prohibit pier construction.

Just past the twin towers is the Washington Pioneer Hall, a 1910 building given to the community by pioneer developer Judge John McGilvra. A plaque in front of the hall also acknowledges the efforts of another pioneer, Loretta Denny, to honor the city's pioneer families.

Across the street from Pioneer Hall is the Madison Park children's play area, featuring "McGilvra's Farm," a collection of stone animal sculptures created by Richard Beyer.

➤Continue down 43rd Avenue East to its intersection with East Madison Street. Ferryboats once debarked from this spot when they crossed Lake Washington to Kirkland. Cars and buses now make the crossing via Evergreen Point Floating Bridge, just north of Madison Park.

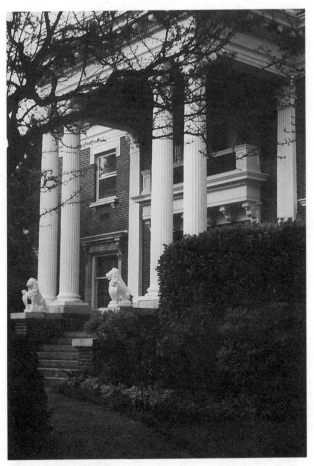

*The Russian Consulate now occupies this historic mansion on East Madison Street.*

➤A block past East Madison Street, at 2012 43rd Avenue East, is the Lake Court Apartments complex. It was designed in the French Provincial Farmhouse style by noted architect Paul Thiry and was built in 1936. The original red-brick Lake Court is now combined with beige, stucco-covered apartments to the north. Together they comprise a unique complex of colorful tiles, turrets, winding staircases, hanging lanterns, and fairy-tale stained glass.

➤Retrace your steps back to East Madison and turn right, into the heart of a commercial district that features high-ticket import, clothing, and specialty shops. The district also features long-established community treasures like a hardware store, bookstore, bakery, wine shop, two taverns, and the Red Apple grocery store, which has been managed by three generations of the same family.

Across the street from the Red Apple—the only fully carpeted supermarket in Seattle—is the Seattle headquarters for the Junior League.

➤Continue on East Madison Street as it heads uphill. The Russian Consulate now occupies the historic mansion at 3726 East Madison. The entrance to Broadmoor Golf and Country Club is at 36th and Madison. Old-timers remember when the circus annually set up tents on a vacant lot at this address.

➤Turn left onto 36th Avenue East, a street bordered on both sides by towering elm trees. You are now entering what is known as Washington Park. The imposing residence at 1117 36th Avenue, described by architects as California Mission Revival, was built in 1909 for vaudevillian Alexander Pantages. Some of the most spectacular theaters in the western United States carried his name and were part of the Pantages vaudeville circuit.

➤Continue up 36th Avenue East, but watch your step. Tree roots have lifted sections of the sidewalk as much as 3 inches, creating plenty of opportunity to trip and fall.

Note the rambling, modernistic estate at the intersection of 36th Avenue and East Ward Street. From the street, you can barely glimpse the expansive formal garden on the second level.

The residence at 808 36th Avenue East, built in 1907 and once known as the Ames House, is now the home of the University of Washington president. The garden-party area in the back looks out on Lake Washington. The residence at 545 36th Avenue East, which features a panel of wooden inlay that stretches across the front, was built as an experimental wood-products house by the Weyerhaeuser Company.

➤Walk down a steep hill on the uneven sidewalk.

➤Turn left onto Lake Washington Boulevard. The crosswalk you see connects the upper and lower campuses of Bush School, a private, preparatory school. On your left at 408 Lake Washington Boulevard is Heffernan House, a Tudor Revival structure built in 1915 that is now a part of the Bush campus.

➤Turn right at a three-way intersection. Street markings are confusing here. Head toward the triangular, yellow sign that reads "Residential Street, 20 m.p.h." Another sign soon identifies the street as Dorffel Drive East.

The houses at 232, 260, and 270 Dorffel Drive are typical of the early construction in this area. To take advantage of their hilltop views, the houses seem to have been put together at random angles, by architects working with life-sized Lincoln logs.

➤Turn right onto East John Street.

➤Walk one block and turn left onto Madrona Place East.

➤Walk another block and turn left onto Denny Way, which becomes Madrona Drive. Continue to the bus turnaround at the bottom of Madrona Drive.

➤Turn right and retrace your steps along the lakeshore back to the starting and finishing point at Madrona Park.

*walk* 10

# Discovery Park

**General location:** About 5 miles northwest of Seattle's business district.

**Special attractions:** Forest pathways, ocean views, nature exhibits.

**Difficulty rating:** Moderate; well-marked paths and trails, one hill.

**Distance:** 4 miles.

**Estimated time:** 2.5 hours.

**Services:** Tourist information center with exhibits, water, and restrooms.

**Restrictions:** Vehicles are prohibited in the park from 11 P.M. to 6 A.M. Leash and scoop laws for pets are enforced. No pets allowed on the beaches or in the ponds or wetland areas. Collecting of any type is prohibited in the park.

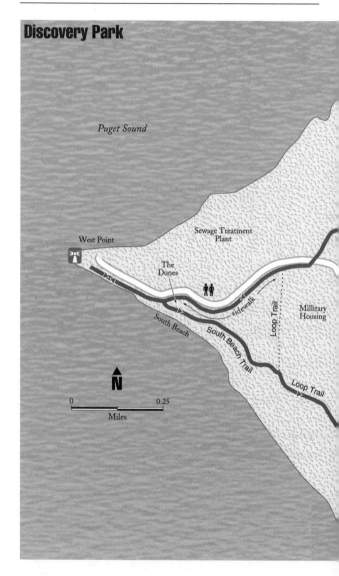

Discovery Park

Puget Sound

West Point

Sewage Treatment
Plant

The
Dunes

South Beach

sidewalk

South Beach Trail

Loop Trail

Military
Housing

Loop Trail

**N**

0                    0.25
Miles

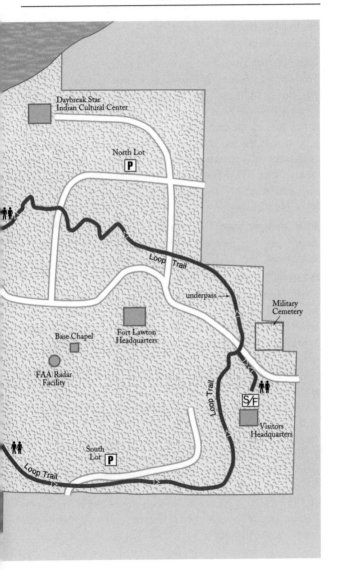

**For more information:** Contact the Discovery Park Visitors' Headquarters.

**Getting started:** From downtown Seattle, drive north on Fourth Avenue, which merges into Denny Way. The road eventually curves right and Denny Way becomes Elliott Avenue. In another mile, Elliott Avenue becomes 15th Avenue West. Take the Dravus Street exit off 15th Avenue West. At the stop sign, turn left to cross the overpass. Turn right onto 20th Avenue West, which merges into Gilman Avenue West. Bear left on West Fort Street, which becomes West Government Way and leads directly to the Discovery Park Visitors' Headquarters.

**Public transportation:** Take Metro Transit Bus 33 north on Fourth Avenue from downtown Seattle to the park headquarters.

**Overview:** In 1938, the U.S. Army offered the citizens of Seattle more than 500 acres of prime, oceanfront property adjacent to expensive homes and just a short drive from the downtown business center. The price tag for the property known as Fort Lawton was one buck. The offer seemed too good to turn down.

But the city did. Officials were concerned about who was going to mow the lawns and trim the hedges of a publicly owned park. Almost three decades later, Seattle got a second chance to acquire the property, this time for free. This time, officials jumped at the chance.

Today Discovery Park is an urban wilderness with more than 150 species of wildlife in its woods and on its beaches. The former army fort is crisscrossed with roads and paths. A 2.8-mile loop trail offers a sampling of all the sights, including native forests, open meadows, and sandy bluffs that overlook Puget Sound.

This is Seattle's largest park and a favorite with hikers, bicyclists, birders, and history buffs.

Captain George Vancouver sailed his ship *Discovery* into Puget Sound in 1792 and gazed up at these forested highlands. By the 1850s, European immigrant farmers were staking claims on the beaches and bluffs. A lighthouse was built on the sand spar called West Point in 1881, and in 1896 the U.S. Army decided it needed a fortification on the high ground overlooking Seattle and the sound.

Thus, construction began on Fort Lawton. Following the Spanish-American War, the Army built corrals and chutes here to handle 700 horses being shipped to the Philippines. During World War II, a million troops passed through the fort. But the long-range mission of the fort was never clearly defined, so the Army decided to deed the land to the city in exchange for a silver dollar.

In 1964, 26 years after that offer was rejected, Fort Lawton was declared surplus property. In 1970, U.S. Senator Henry Jackson and President Richard Nixon drafted the Fort Lawton Bill, which later became a model for public acquisition of surplus military sites.

Several special-interest groups wanted a piece of the real estate when Congress created Discovery Park. Bernie White Bear waged one of the most energetic campaigns on behalf of Northwest Indians. Seventeen acres were subsequently leased to the Native Americans, and in 1977 Daybreak Star Indian Cultural Center was built in one of the most scenic parts of the park.

A federal military cemetery, an Army church, and some other relics of the fort still occupy the grounds, including some homes occupied by military personnel currently stationed in the area. The officers' quarters above the parade ground, completed in 1904, is on the National Register of Historic Places.

Extending beyond Discovery Park is the neighborhood of Seattle known as Magnolia Bluff. The name should actually be Madrona Bluff. Navy geographer George Davidson is responsible for the error. In 1897, he mistakenly identified the native madrona trees as magnolias.

With views of Puget Sound and the Olympic Mountains beyond, Magnolia Bluff is a prestigious address in Seattle, even if the federal government could not sell it for a buck.

# the walk

Before starting your walk, pick up a map at the Discovery Park Visitors' Headquarters. Construction on this facility, which also houses the Environmental Education Center, began in 1986. The center features a variety of interesting family-oriented displays highlighting the flora and fauna of the park. Restrooms are provided, and you can obtain informational pamphlets from the ranger at the front desk. On weekends, shuttle buses run from the visitors' headquarters to South Beach for those with limited mobility.

➤Walk straight out the main entrance of the visitors' headquarters and follow the sign on the left that directs you to the Discovery Park Loop Trail.

➤At the top of a small rise are three paths. Take the path that leads straight ahead to an underpass under one of the park roads. The loop trail will soon cross one and then another of the paved roads in the park, built for military use but now almost free of traffic.

The loop trail passes a giant maple tree with a quintuple trunk rising toward the forest canopy. The path crosses two more paved roads. A right turn down the second road leads in 200 yards to the Daybreak Star Indian Cultural Center.

You may choose to make a side trip to the center. It is open to the public but is primarily a meeting facility for the Northwest tribes.

➤Continue on the marked loop trail. You will pass a residential area that once housed military personnel at Fort Lawton. There is a crossing sign where the loop trail meets one of the park's main, public-access roads.

➤Turn right onto the sidewalk that borders the access road. This leads you downhill to the beach. Keep an eye out for bald eagles, which nest in this area. In fact, this is generally regarded as one of the top bird-watching areas in King County.

The beach to the distant right of the walkway is the site of the West Point Sewage Treatment Plant. You will not notice its function if the wind is blowing from the south.

➤Walk another quarter-mile along the tree-lined road and you will reach restrooms. From this point on, the sidewalk continues on the opposite side of the road.

➤Take the path at the bottom of the hill that connects with the sidewalk. This route leads toward the West Point Light Station. Built in 1881, this functioning lighthouse is the oldest in the Seattle area. It is maintained by the U.S. Coast Guard.

Watch for seals and sea lions in the waters off West Point. Paths run from the lighthouse to the right along the beach and past the sewage-treatment plant. Or you can retrace your steps and explore the South Beach area, where there are fascinating tide pools and a variety of sandy beaches, rocky beaches, and mud flats.

➤A quarter-mile from the lighthouse along South Beach, look for a marker leading you to a trailhead for the South Beach Trail.

➤Head uphill on this trail. As the sign indicates, the path connects South Beach with the Discovery Park Loop Trail. The route is fairly steep, but the trail is well maintained and there are observation platforms where you can catch your breath.

➤The South Beach Trail rejoins the Discovery Park Loop Trail near an area of small sand hills known as the Dunes. This is a great place for a picnic because you are at the top of a bluff that overlooks the water and islands of Puget

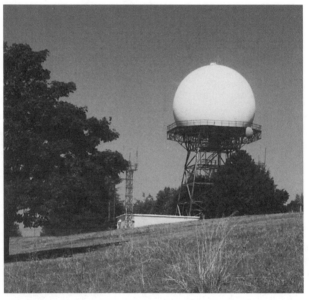

*This giant "golf ball" is actually a radar facility used by the Federal Aviation Administration to control air traffic.*

### How High the Sky?

Seattle was once known as "The City of Seven Hills." Granted, Rome probably holds the copyright on that title. And if Seattle ever did have that many prominent peaks, it does not anymore.

In an attempt to create a new and relatively level city center, city officials in 1897 initiated a project to remove Denny Hill. City Engineer R. H. Thomson directed the project, which involved using dynamite, heavy equipment, and millions of gallons of water pumped from Lake Union through high-pressure hoses to transform Denny Hill into the Denny Regrade.

Initially, the project created a sea of mud. Today, Denny Regrade is one of the fastest growing residential areas in the city. But it is no longer a hill.

What were the other sites referred to in "The City of Seven Hills?" According to one source, they were Queen Anne Hill, Magnolia Bluff, First Hill, Capitol Hill, Beacon Hill, and Profanity Hill, more commonly known as Yesler.

Some modern historians say that Seattle never deserved the title. They claim that Seattle did not have seven hills when the city limits were more restricted. Now, they say, Seattle has more than seven.

Apparently, one geographical fact has been established. According to the Seattle Engineering Department, the highest point in Seattle—512 feet above sea level—is at the foot of a water tower at 35th Avenue Southwest and Myrtle Street in West Seattle. Nobody was really aware of that precise statistic when they named that district Highpoint.

Sound. Harbor seals frequent the beach below. On a typical summer Sunday, you might see 50 to 100 sailboats, two or three ferries, a freighter or two from the Far East, possibly the catamarán *Victoria Clipper* headed for Canada, and some scattered kayakers. The closest landmass across the sound is Bainbridge Island, and the snowcapped Olympic Mountains loom beyond. On clear days, Mount Rainier is also visible from this point.

➤Continue on the loop trail, which is marked by logs laid end to end on the bluff side of the path. The giant white "golf ball" on your left is a Federal Aviation Administration radar facility used to control air traffic within a 200-mile radius of Sea-Tac International Airport.

➤The loop trail passes restrooms and a drinking fountain and then continues on to the south park entrance and parking lot. Markers indicate where it continues from the parking lot.

➤When you come to a junction of the trail and a road, follow the trail to the right. The road dead-ends at a barrier. The loop trail continues along the park boundary and then veers left into the heart of the park.

➤A path cuts off to the right and leads downhill, but ignore this route and continue straight ahead through groves of maples, alders, and some tall evergreens. The path crosses a paved road.

➤Turn right just past the paved road at the sign identifying the route back to the visitors' headquarters and parking lot.

*walk* 11

# Woodland Park Zoo

**General location:** About 4 miles north of the city center, just west of Washington Highway 99.

**Special attractions:** Zoo, food concessions, bookstore, and gift shop.

**Difficulty rating:** Easy; paved walkways and dirt paths.

**Distance:** 1.25 miles.

**Estimated time:** 1.5 hours.

**Services:** Food booths, restrooms, wheelchair and stroller rentals.

**Restrictions:** No smoking on secondary paths, at viewpoints, or in zoo buildings. No pets except seeing-eye dogs. Do not feed the animals, and do not tap on glass or otherwise stress the animals.

127

# Woodland Park Zoo

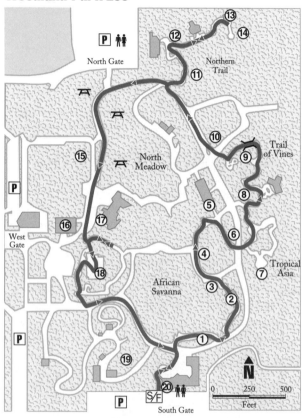

1 Giraffe Pole
2 African Bird Enclosure
3 Hippo Pond
4 Giraffe House
5 Lions
6 Hyenas
7 Thai Village
8 Tapirs, Siamang Lesser Apes
9 Orangutans
10 Raptor Center
11 Wolves
12 Bears, Otters
13 Bald Eagles
14 Elk
15 Pony Rides
16 Rain Forest Cafe
17 Gorillas
18 Tropical Rain Forest
19 Family Farm
20 Zoo Store

**For more information:** Contact Woodland Park Zoo.

**Getting started:** From the city center, take Interstate 5 north to the Northeast 50th Street exit (Exit 169). Drive west on Northeast 50th Street to the south gate of the zoo, at North 50th Street and Fremont Avenue.

**Public transportation:** Board Metro Transit Bus 5, which goes north from Third Avenue and Pike Street in downtown Seattle. Exit at the zoo's west gate, at North 55th Street and Phinney Avenue North. Follow the path along the zoo fence in a counterclockwise direction to reach the south gate.

**Overview:** In the past two decades, numerous awards from the American Zoo and Aquarium Association have established Woodland Park as one of the most progressive and humane zoos in the United States.

One of the few dissenting opinions was registered by Kiki the gorilla, and he voted with his feet. Kiki used a tree branch to bust out of his exhibit in 1980, but he may have had good reason to run away from home. The zoo had acquired a female gorilla named Timba for breeding purposes, and even folks with little expertise in the matter considered Kiki's prospective bride devoid of all feminine graces.

At that time, it was almost impossible for a captive gorilla to escape what might be described as an "arranged marriage." In most zoos, the primates were housed behind steel bars and concrete. However, Kiki occupied an open-air exhibit space—the conception of a citizen's task force created in the 1970s. These far-sighted planners had envisioned a zoo with savannas, a tropical rain forest, desert regions, and a "Northern Trail" featuring wolves, bears, eagles, and other creatures of the Northwest. They thought their concept would keep zoo visitors from feeling like peeping Toms, catching furtive glances of captive animals. Rather, visitors would be "immersed" in the animal world as they strolled past grasslands populated by giraffes, zebras, and springboks.

The conversion of Woodland Park Zoo began in 1976. More than $50 million was acquired in 1985, mainly through a bond issue passed by King County voters. Planning for future projects continues today.

The origins of the Seattle zoo extend back to the beginning of the 20th century. The city purchased the 200-acre estate of Guy Carlton Phinney from his widow for $500 cash and assumption of the mortgage. The Woodland Park Zoo opened in April 1904 with a couple of bears, a few birds, and some deer and elk. Development proceeded at the pace of a three-toed sloth. The original bear pits and cages were not replaced until 1965, when a Woodland Park Zoological Society was created to organize planning and fundraising. The zoo now has 1,000 animals, a small army of volunteers, and sophisticated education, research, and breeding programs. It has come a long way since a resident gorilla tried unsuccessfully to opt out of "The Dating Game."

Viewing tip: The animals tend to be liveliest in the morning, just after the zoo has opened.

# the walk

➤Enter the zoo's south gate and walk straight ahead toward the sign reading "African Savanna." From the savanna overlook, you can often see giraffes and zebras roaming the unfenced grasslands.

➤Follow the sign to the right marked "More Animals." Next to the path on the right is a pole showing the average height of giraffes. Look to the left and note the bales of hay tied into the yokes of trees at a feeding height of about 17 feet.

➤Turn left as the savanna overlook trail joins a paved path

leading toward the lion exhibits. Another savanna overlook in a boulder field on the left offers glimpses of zebras, giraffes, and springboks.

➤Enter the enclosure containing birds of the African savanna. Note the pear-shaped nests of the southern masked weavers. Males attract their mates by hanging upside down from the nests, flapping their wings, and singing loudly.

➤Exit the bird exhibit and walk to the viewpoint on the left, which overlooks the hippo pool. On warm days, you are liable to see nothing more than a portion of the submerged hippos' backs. Be patient; they come up for breath every five minutes. The hippos used to be at their liveliest the day after Halloween, when a few leftover pumpkins were tossed into the pool, much like an apple-dunking contest for kids. The practice went on for several years but finally was discontinued. Like a lot of trick-and-treaters, the hippos woke up the next morning with tummy aches.

➤Just after you pass a bronze statue of sleeping hippos, note the giraffe house on your right. It is here, where the public is not allowed to intrude, that the majestic animals spend their "quiet time" at the zoo.

➤Walk straight ahead at the intersection of two paths. This will lead you to a viewpoint from which you may spot lions basking on bare rocks.

➤Retrace your steps back to the intersection and turn left at the sign pointing to "Tropical Asia." This path leads past another lion overlook and a videotape showing savanna animals in their natural habitat. The path will take you past the cages of spotted hyenas, on your left.

➤As you circle right on the path and head downhill, note two signs. One of them points to the elephant barns and a "Thai Village," where working-elephant demonstrations are regularly presented.

➤Our route goes to the left on the path marked "Trail of Vines." You will pass giant pythons and animals like the western tufted deer, Malayan tapir, lion-tailed macaque, and siamang lesser ape. When they are in the mood, the baboon-like siamangs, natives of Sumatra, emit hoots and howls that can be heard a half-mile away.

➤Just past the siamang area is an indoor-outdoor complex with a picturesque waterfall that houses the orangutans. Zoo officials kept a close watch on the orangutans when this exhibit first opened, for fear the long-armed vine swingers might soar or scamper right over the walls. Fortunately, none did. Woodland Park Zoo is conducting extensive research into the habits of these great apes.

➤Cross the wooden bridge leading away from the orangutan exhibit and bear right toward the Raptor Center. Owls, falcons, and other raptors are usually sitting on perches here, and a handler is often present to answer questions or conduct flight demonstrations.

➤Beyond the Raptor Center, follow the signs directing you to the "Northern Trail" exhibit. A large sign marks the entrance. The paved path goes downhill and past some artificially created caves, which are irresistible to small children.

You might spot wolves on your immediate right. To the left, on a small loop trail look for porcupines high up in the trees. An indoor exhibit uses photographs and recordings to describe the sights and sounds of the great Northwest.

➤Continue down the hill and look to your left for bears. Sometimes you will spot them digging into a log. At other times they will be indoors, behind thick glass walls, in a cave, or cavorting in a fish-filled pond.

In another glass enclosure, river otters streak through the water and dart between submerged tree branches. They of-

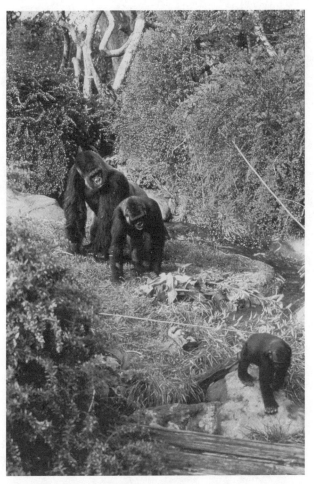

*The gorillas at the Woodland Park Zoo have room to roam in this naturally inviting outdoor enclosure. Woodland Park photo by Ian Dewar*

ten seem to be playing hide-and-seek with the fascinated young children on the other side of the glass.

➤Past the bear and otter exhibits are viewpoints overlooking an enormous bald eagle nest and, farther down the path, an elk herd.

➤Retrace your steps out of the Northern Trail exhibit and back to the main path circling the zoo.

➤Turn right onto the loop trail. It will take you past the north gate, and then it curves left past a pony-ride concession to the entrance of the Rain Forest Café, a collection of fast-food counters with indoor and outdoor dining.

➤Take a left turn just past the entrance to the Rain Forest Café and follow the signs to the gorilla viewing area. There are usually two gorilla groups on display. Although they have been provided with a natural outdoor habitat, they seem to enjoy sitting next to the glass walls for the best views of the passing tourists.

➤Retrace your steps back toward the Rain Forest Café and then follow the sign leading you to the "Tropical Rain Forest." The indoor exhibit features a colorful collection of ocelots, tropical fish, birds, poison-dart frogs, and tree boas.

➤Continue on into the "Rain Forest Canopy," a sort of biosphere for wild birds.

➤Turn left onto the connector path when you exit the Rain Forest Canopy and follow the signs to the "Family Farm" and south gate. The Family Farm, which features barnyard animals and a petting corral, is an optional loop off the main zoo trail.

➤Our walk turns left onto the main zoo trail just a few hundred feet from the starting and finishing point at the south gate. Here you will find restrooms, water fountains, and the Woodland Park Zoo Store.

*walk* 12

# Green Lake

 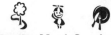  

**General location:** North Seattle, just east of Washington Highway 99 (Aurora Avenue).

**Special attractions:** Shops, restaurants, lake views, fishing, boating, swimming, wading pool, playgrounds.

**Difficulty rating:** Easy; flat, entirely on paved path.

**Distance:** 2.9 miles.

**Estimated time:** 1.25 hours.

**Services:** Drinking fountains and restrooms at the small-craft center where the walk begins; restaurants and boat and roller-skate rentals are located at various points around the lake.

**Restrictions:** The path around Green Lake has designated lanes for "heels" and "wheels." Walkers, runners, and baby strollers are restricted to the inside lane, while bicyclists and skaters are restricted to the outside. It is recommended that

## Green Lake

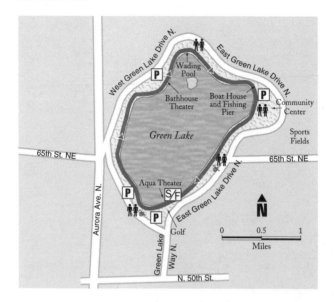

walkers proceed in a clockwise direction around the lake. Leash and scoop laws for pets are enforced.

**For more information:** Contact the Seattle Parks Department.

**Getting started:** From downtown Seattle, head north on the Alaskan Way Viaduct. It parallels the waterfront. The viaduct becomes WA 99, also known as Aurora Avenue North. Take the 50th Street exit off Aurora and drive east (to your right). Turn left onto Green Lake Way. Watch carefully because you must turn left in about three blocks onto poorly marked Green Lake Avenue North, and you will miss it if you are traveling too fast. The left turn takes you past a par-three golf course, on your right. Just past the golf course, park in one of the free Green Lake parking areas, on either side of the road.

**Public transportation:** Board Metro Transit Bus 6 and head north on Third Avenue. Get off at the Green Lake Pitch and Putt golf course, at the south end of the lake.

**Overview:** Marathon runners in training, toddlers in strollers, and walkers of all ages share the paths around Green Lake with dogs on leashes, inline skaters, kids on three-wheelers, and serious bicyclists astride $2,000 Italian imports. On busy weekends, the scene sometimes resembles 500 squirrels in an enormous revolving cage, but major collisions between "heels" and "wheels" are rare.

In the 1880s, this area was more of a remote swamp than a lake, and it was mainly known as the permanent haunt of Erhart Saifraid, alias Green Lake John. He cooked meals over an open fire and sometimes shook his fist at gawking visitors from downtown Seattle.

Today a theater occupies a bathhouse on the lakefront. The lake itself is ringed by anglers and dotted with sailboats, kayaks, and racing shells. Nearby are soccer fields, softball diamonds, a par-three golf course, and one of the city's most pleasant residential areas.

As one of the signs posted at the lake reminds visitors, the area would probably be known today as Green Marsh or Green Meadows if the city had not taken corrective measures to create and preserve the lake. Dredging, water diversion from nearby reservoirs, and the elimination of one feeder stream were required to create the lake you see today.

This walk begins near a structure once known as the Green Lake Aqua Theater. A group of synchronized swimmers called the Aqua Dears once kicked up their heels in the frigid waters of the lake. Clown divers executed acrobatic flips off the twin diving towers. Bands played and singers

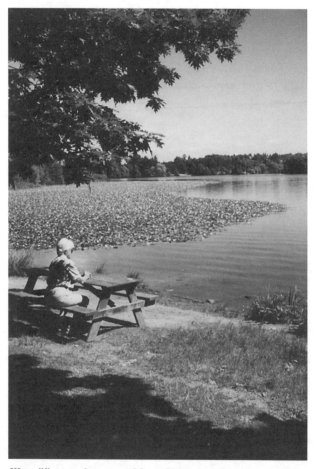

*Water lilies crowd a corner of Green Lake near this popular picnic spot.*

performed on the stage that was a part of the Aqua Theater complex. In the 1950s and 1960s, thousands of spectators trooped to the lake carrying blankets and beverages. It is often cool at the lake after sundown, even in July and August. Or maybe the fans needed blankets because of the goose bumps they got watching the Aqua Dears emerge dripping wet from the icy water, into the chill wind.

The Aqua Dears and divers are gone, but they imbued Green Lake with a sense of health and fitness that is still apparent today.

# the walk

➤Begin walking clockwise around the lake from the parking area at the site of the former Green Lake Aqua Theater. Almost immediately you pass the Green Lake Small-Craft Center, headquarters for rowing crews and for sailing and canoeing enthusiasts. There are accessible restrooms and drinking fountains at the center.

➤After a quarter-mile, the trail parallels busy Aurora Avenue North. Look left across Aurora where the trail turns to see the Twin Teepees restaurant, a longtime neighborhood fixture.

➤The path circles right past some tennis courts. Often, rowing crews will pause at this part of the lake before sprinting back to the small-craft center. You may hear the rowing coaches barking instructions through battery-powered megaphones.

The Bathhouse Theater on your right, built in 1928 and since remodeled, has been the site of year-round legitimate theater. A swimming area with floats and a slide is located behind the theater. Drinking fountains are outside the theater

**of interest**

## The Twin Teepees

No plaques indicate the historical significance of the Twin Teepees, a favorite dining spot for many Green Lake visitors and residents. But there probably should be something hanging in the Twin Teepees kitchen, once the temporary hangout of a gastronomical genius-in-waiting.

The late Walter Clark not only operated a chain of quality restaurants in Seattle, but he also served as director of the National Restaurant Association during the 1940s. At one of the association conventions, he met another energetic restaurateur who had fallen upon hard times. The fellow operated a highway diner in Kentucky, but wartime gas rationing had slowed traffic and put Clark's acquaintance out of business.

Clark offered his new friend a temporary job as cook at one of his downtown Seattle restaurants. But the other workers complained that when business was at a peak, the new guy was no help. He was usually off in some corner measuring out different herbs and spices, they said. Finally, one of the other chefs sent a note to Clark.

"Get this clown out of the way," the chef suggested.

To keep peace in the kitchen, Clark moved his friend to the Twin Teepees, where the man's fascination with herbs and spices continued. After 10 months, the man decided to move back to Kentucky, where he opened a new restaurant featuring a special recipe.

You guessed it. The chef began calling himself Colonel Sanders, and his specialty—Kentucky Fried Chicken—made dining history.

The menu at the Twin Teepees does not feature the Colonel's finger-licking chicken.

entrance. Just past the theater, note the photographs showing scenes of Green Lake from the era of trolley cars to the present.

➤Between the theater and a children's wading pool, look off to the left to note two potential places to stop for lunch: Duke's Chowder House and Six Degrees, a restaurant and pub. There are also coffee shops, bakeries, and ice cream shops along this stretch of East Green Lake Drive North.

There are restrooms adjacent to the wading pool.

The boat rental complex is the center of greatest activity on the lake. Visitors can rent pedal boats, sailboats, windsurfing gear, and canoes. There is also a fishing pier and a swimming area with lifeguards posted during the summer. Drinks and snacks are available at stands adjacent to the path in this area.

➤Just past the boating center are two large, cream-colored structures that comprise the Green Lake Community Center, where recreation classes and activities are held. On the left just past the community center are large fields where softball, touch football, rugby, and soccer are played, depending on the season. Look for bald eagles in the tallest trees around the lake and particularly on the small island near the north shore.

➤At the intersection of East Green Lake Drive North and 65th Street Northeast, on your left, there are restrooms and drinking fountains. Ahead and to your left is the par-three golf course and beyond it the old Aqua Theater, where you start and finish this walk.

*walk* 13

# Seward Park

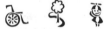

**General location:** On Bailey Peninsula in Lake Washington, about 6 miles southeast of central Seattle, adjacent to Interstate 90 and Lacey V. Morrow Memorial Bridge.

**Special attractions:** Old-growth forest, bird watching, nautical views, swimming beaches, picnic areas.

**Difficulty rating:** Easy to moderate, depending upon whether you choose the short or long route; flat, almost entirely on paved paths or sidewalks.

**Distance:** 2.5 or 6.5 miles, depending on route.

**Estimated time:** 1.5 hours for short route, 3 hours for long route.

**Services:** Restrooms and water at the entrance to Seward Park and at Sayres Park.

# Seward Park

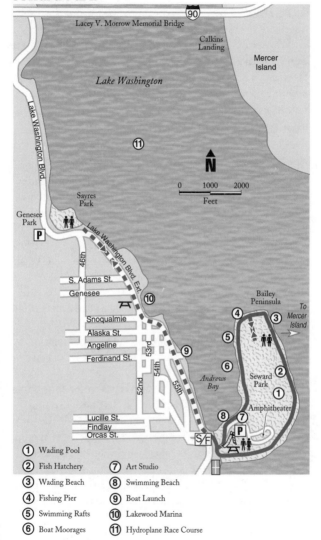

Lacey V. Morrow Memorial Bridge

Calkins Landing

Mercer Island

*Lake Washington*

⑪

**N**

| 0 | 1000 | 2000 |

Feet

Sayres Park

Genesee Park

**P**

Lake Washington Blvd.

46th

Lake Washington Blvd. Ext.

S. Adams St.

Genesee

⑩

Snoqualmie

Alaska St.

Angeline

Ferdinand St.

53rd

⑨

52nd

54th

55th

*Andrews Bay*

Bailey Peninsula

④

⑤

⑥

To Mercer Island →

Seward Park

②

①

Lucille St.

Findlay

Orcas St.

S/F

⑧ ⑦

**P**

Amphitheater

① Wading Pool

② Fish Hatchery

③ Wading Beach

④ Fishing Pier

⑤ Swimming Rafts

⑥ Boat Moorages

⑦ Art Studio

⑧ Swimming Beach

⑨ Boat Launch

⑩ Lakewood Marina

⑪ Hydroplane Race Course

143

**For more information:** Contact the Seattle Parks Department.

**Getting started:** Drive south on Interstate 5 from downtown Seattle. Leave I-5 at Exit 163-A and bear left on Columbian Way. Drive 1.5 miles and turn left onto Beacon Avenue South. Turn left onto South Orcas Street and drive to the lakefront. Turn right onto Lake Washington Boulevard, and almost immediately you will see the Seward Park sign and entrance. Parking is free.

**Public transportation:** Board Metro Transit Bus 39 at designated stops on Second Avenue and travel south. Get off at Seward Park Avenue South and South Orcas Street.

**Overview:** In 1903, the Olmsted firm of landscape architects presented its plan for a series of public parks in Seattle linked by greenbelts like Lake Washington Boulevard. Seward Park, at the south end of the boulevard, was not included in the master plan for a very good reason. The 277-acre tract was an island until 1916, when the opening of the Lake Washington Ship Canal lowered the water level of the lake enough to expose a connecting stem of land, creating what is now Bailey Peninsula (better known locally as the Seward Park peninsula).

The loop trail around the peninsula is bordered on one side by old-growth forest and on the other by Lake Washington, with views of South Seattle and Mercer Island.

Cedar waxwings flock to Seward Park in the springtime, attracted by the crop of serviceberries. Red-headed nuthatches are commonly seen in the Douglas-firs. Pacific tree frogs live in the vine maples. Towhees and woodpeckers abound. And when the native blue violets are in bloom, great spangled fritillary butterflies put on a spectacular display.

In 1929, the first of 3,500 Japanese cherry trees was planted in Seattle by former Premier Wakatsuki and Admiral and

Madame Takarabe, who arrived here with a fleet of Japanese naval training ships. A plaque next to a Taiko-Gata lantern at the entrance to Seward Park notes that the flowering trees "manifested the gratitude of the people of Yokohama for the assistance given them by the citizens of Seattle on the occasion of the disastrous earthquake of 1923." Most of these trees line Lake Washington Boulevard, beginning here at the park.

# the walk

The basic walk consists of the 2.5-mile loop around Seward Park. When this route is completed, you can decide whether to extend the walk another 4 miles by following the lakeshore to Sayres Park and back for more nautical views and glimpses of the lifestyles and homes of lakefront residents.

➤From the Seward Park entrance, walk past the children's playground and a covered outdoor dining pavilion identified as Stove and Picnic Area No. 1. Continue on toward a paved path that runs along the shore of Lake Washington.

➤Turn left onto the path, which loops around the park. The area you see across the water and to your right is South Seattle. The landmass directly ahead is Mercer Island.

➤The path turns left and widens into a boulevard lined with weeping willows, madronas, and western redcedars. You will be sharing the path with bicyclists, but signs instruct them to warn pedestrians using bell or voice when passing.

The waters to your right are popular with water-skiers, and wetsuits have transformed this form of recreation into a year-round activity.

If you brought along binoculars, you now have excellent views of Mercer Island beach homes and boathouses on your right. According to a Duwamish Indian legend, an evil spirit once resided on Lake Washington's only island. Author Jack London and friends once rowed from Seattle to Mercer Island, with muffled oars, to attend an illegal bare-knuckles fight in the woods. Later, Mercer Island became a summer retreat accessible by ferryboat. With the construction in 1940 of the Lacey V. Morrow Memorial Bridge, which links Seattle with the island, Mercer Island lost its isolation and gained a reputation as one of the richest residential communities in the Northwest. It is now the home of such financial giants as Paul Allen, co-founder of Microsoft.

Anglers on the lakeshore in Seward Park cast their lures in the direction of Mercer Island. Others fish from boats anchored on this east side of the peninsula.

➤Watch on your left for a small waterfall linking what was once a fish hatchery with the lake. The hatchery grounds are now off-limits to visitors. A stone bridge above the waterfall, erected in 1934 by a local sports council, is still visible from the road.

Through the tunnel of trees ahead, you will soon see the Lacey V. Morrow Memorial Bridge, one of two floating spans across Lake Washington. Notice the spot where the bridge reaches Mercer Island. Just this side of it, C. C. Calkins built a three-story resort hotel in the 1880s. It featured storybook towers, a grand ballroom, a series of verandas overlooking 25 fountains, a manicured lawn, and a giant greenhouse. There were bathhouses, swimming beaches, and a dock where President Benjamin Harrison arrived by steamer in 1891. The Calkins Hotel was a victim of an economic depression and later burned to the ground.

➤Follow the path as it turns left near the north end of the Seward Park peninsula. The floating bridge is now fully visible, along with the skyscrapers of downtown Seattle. Because of the views and a sandy beach, this is a popular wading and picnicking area.

➤Just past the restrooms, there is a dirt path off to the left. It enters the forest and climbs through the woods to the upper level of Seward Park. If you want to leave the beach path to explore this impressive forest of old-growth trees, this is probably the best trail. Several trails crisscross the summit of the hill, but many of them lead to dead ends. So return to the beach path by this same route.

➤As you continue around the north end of the peninsula, note across the water a small marina located on Lake Washington Boulevard. It is usually filled to capacity with sailboats and cabin cruisers.

➤The beach path continues to turn left, and you are now headed directly toward the Seward Park entrance. On your right as you make this final turn is the Rev. U. G. Murphy Fishing Pier. Beyond the pier, in Andrews Bay, you may see 30 or more boats anchored for a weekend stay in protected waters. Boaters and picnickers from the beach meet on hot summer days atop a series of fishing rafts anchored offshore. Water-lily pads block access from the shore to the rafts in some areas.

A road to the left leads uphill from the beach path to an amphitheater where concerts are occasionally scheduled.

➤Continuing on the beach path, you come to a small brick building that serves as an art studio. Workbenches occupy the main floor, and a small gallery, open to visitors, is on the second level. The beach just behind the studio is yet another popular swimming site.

➤Just beyond the art studio, you can see the playground and the Seward Park entrance. You have walked a total of 2.5 miles and can end your walk here. Or you may choose to

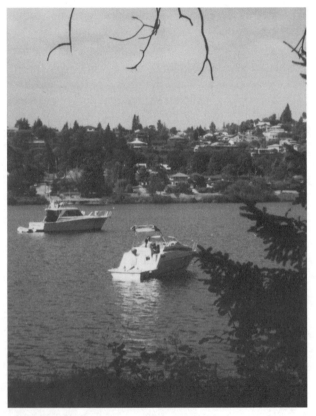

*Pleasure craft jockey for position on Andrews Bay, just offshore from Seward Park.*

extend your walk by continuing for 2 miles along Lake Washington Boulevard South to Stan Sayres Memorial Park.

➤If you choose to continue, turn right out of the park onto Lake Washington Boulevard South. The boulevard, lined with Japanese cherry trees, is a part of Mount Baker Park.

Homes along the parkway present a display of contrasting architecture, including Olde English, California Beach Modern, and Northwest ramblers. On the east side of the street, a launching area for small boats is located at the intersection with Ferdinand Street.

➤Continue on for a closer look at the Lakewood Marina, which you first glimpsed from Seward Park. There are tables and picnic sites with sweeping views where Lake Washington Boulevard intersects with South Adams Street and again at 50th Avenue South. The beaches from here all the way to the floating bridge are lined with hundreds of thousands of spectators the first Sunday in August when the unlimited hydroplanes stage their annual regatta on Lake Washington. The center of this unique sporting event is Sayres Park, the turnaround for this extended walk. During race week, the big powerboats occupy both sides of the finger piers and are hoisted into and out of the water by construction cranes. The rest of the year, Sayres Park is a headquarters for rowing and sailing classes. Sayres Park also includes ramps for launching pleasure boats, ample parking, and restrooms.

Across Lake Washington Boulevard from Sayres Park is Genesee Park, which has playgrounds and picnic facilities.

➤Turn around at this Sayres-Genesee recreation complex and retrace your steps along Lake Washington Boulevard back to the starting and finishing point at the Seward Park entrance.

**of interest**

### Thunderboats

This pastoral site along Lake Washington is home to cedar waxwings, tree frogs, spangled butterflies, and the red-headed nuthatch. But for one weekend each year, the birds and bugs take second billing to Blue Angels and Thunderboats. The latter, the fastest race boats in the world, make ear-splitting, 200-mile-an-hour sprints around a course that runs between Seward Park and the Lacey V. Morrow Memorial Bridge.

Seafair, an unlimited hydroplane regatta that generally takes place the first Sunday of August, is Seattle's answer to the Kentucky Derby and Indy 500. The daylong event often draws crowds of 300,000 or more. Between heats, the Navy's acrobatic team of jet pilots, the Blue Angels, often performs over the lake.

Before there were any major-league sports teams in Seattle, local kids traded hydroplane buttons, towed toy boats behind their bicycles, and swapped stories about their favorite racing heroes. They recalled the day Wild Bill Cantrell lost control of his hydroplane, Gale IV, and after skidding to a stop, found himself in the middle of a garden party at a home on Lakeside Avenue South. They remembered when the late Bill Muncey lost the rudder, and his hydroplane rammed and sank a Coast Guard patrol boat anchored near Seward Park.

Old-timers remember when the Slo-mo-shun boats would disappear shortly before the start of a race. Then they would come thundering underneath the west span of the floating bridge and past sputtering rival boats in a hair-raising tactic that has since been outlawed.

The Slo-mos, as they were known then, were owned by Seattle millionaire Stan Sayres. The park that bears his name still serves as the pit area on the day each year when the Blue Angels and Thunderboats drown out the songbirds.

*walk* 14

# Campus

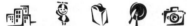

**General location:** About 4 miles north of the city center.

**Special attractions:** Architecturally acclaimed university campus and shopping district, Burke Museum of Natural History and Culture, Henry Art Gallery.

**Difficulty rating:** Easy; flat, on paths and sidewalks, except for two moderate stairways.

**Distance:** 3 miles.

**Estimated time:** 1.5 hours.

**Services:** Several restaurants; cafes, drinking water, and accessible bathrooms in Burke Museum, Henry Gallery, and Student Union.

**Restrictions:** Leash and scoop laws for pets are enforced. The Henry Gallery is closed Mondays and on some national

# Campus

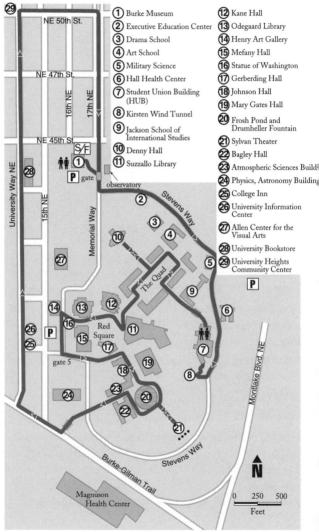

1 Burke Museum
2 Executive Education Center
3 Drama School
4 Art School
5 Military Science
6 Hall Health Center
7 Student Union Building (HUB)
8 Kirsten Wind Tunnel
9 Jackson School of International Studies
10 Denny Hall
11 Suzzallo Library
12 Kane Hall
13 Odegaard Library
14 Henry Art Gallery
15 Mefany Hall
16 Statue of Washington
17 Gerberding Hall
18 Johnson Hall
19 Mary Gates Hall
20 Frosh Pond and Drumheller Fountain
21 Sylvan Theater
22 Bagley Hall
23 Atmospheric Sciences Building
24 Physics, Astronomy Building
25 College Inn
26 University Information Center
27 Allen Center for the Visual Arts
28 University Bookstore
29 University Heights Community Center

holidays. Campus buildings are generally open from 8 A.M. to 5 P.M.

**For more information:** Contact the University of Washington, Burke Museum, or Henry Gallery.

**Getting started:** Head north from downtown Seattle on Interstate 5. Take the 45th Street exit and turn right onto 17th Avenue Northeast. Follow 17th to the University of Washington entrance booth and Burke Museum parking lot.

**Public transportation:** Board northbound Metro Transit Bus 70 on Third Avenue in downtown Seattle. Get off at 15th Avenue Northeast and Northeast 45th Street and walk two blocks to 17th Avenue Northeast.

**Overview:** The scientists, philosophers, historians, and Nobel laureates who occupy positions of prominence on the University of Washington campus owe at least a tip of their mortarboards to Prince Albert the Talking Horse and La Belle Zamona's belly dancers. Big Al and Zamona were midway stars of the Alaska-Yukon-Pacific Exposition of 1909, an event that transformed the university's image locally and nationally. But the biggest celebrity that summer was William Howard Taft—even though he never actually appeared in person. Back in Washington, D.C., the president pressed a golden telegraph key to flick on the lights of the exposition, which attracted representatives of 26 countries to the opulent buildings and grounds landscaped by the Olmsted Brothers of New York.

Founded in 1861, the UW located its first campus in what is now the center of Seattle's business district. It moved to its present location in 1895, putting it a long streetcar ride away from downtown. There were no paved streets or sewers in the area, and the campus had few buildings that could not have easily been converted into chicken sheds.

The Alaska-Yukon-Pacific Exposition provided the $10 million needed to transform that rural site. Expo buildings and grounds provided a foundation for what has become one of the most picturesque campuses in the West.

Today, classrooms are located in a mix of modern and neo-Gothic buildings on 694 acres of parklike grounds adjoining Lake Washington and Portage Bay. Some 35,000 students are enrolled in more than 100 academic disciplines at 16 major schools and colleges. The UW work force numbers 17,000, and the school operates both the University of Washington Medical Center and Harborview Medical Center.

And although school historians do not dwell upon the point, it all started, in a way, with Prince Albert the Talking Horse and La Belle Zamona.

# the walk

➤If you arrive on foot, enter the campus through the gate at 45th Street and 17th Avenue Northeast. A plaque at the entrance is dedicated to university men killed in World War I. Pick up a campus map at the guard booth, but be forewarned that few of the roadways and even fewer of the paths identified on the map are marked with signs or directional arrows.

➤If you are driving, tell the attendant at the booth that you would like to park in the lot at the Burke Museum of Natural History and Culture. You can visit the museum before or after the walk.

Just across Memorial Way from the Burke Museum is the University Observatory, established in 1892. The guard booth, museum, and observatory are all located on Memorial Way.

**The Burke Museum**

• A 15-million-year-old rhino skeleton found in Blue Lake near Coulee City.

• A 25-million-year-old baleen whale fossil discovered near Physt.

• A 70-million-year-old elasmosaur from Nanaimo, British Columbia.

• The 140-million-year-old remains of a flesh-eating *Allosaurus,* the only dinosaur skeleton found in the Northwest.

These are just four of the 3 million artifacts and specimens in the collections of the Burke Museum of Natural History and Culture on the University of Washington campus.

The museum was founded in 1879 by a group of men who called themselves the Young Naturalist Society. That organization has since evolved into a museum society that extends to visitors the opportunity to "Go back to a time when dinosaurs roamed—and giant marine reptiles ruled the seas."

The Burke has two permanent exhibits. One highlights the 500-million-year history of the Pacific Northwest and offers children—and their parents—the opportunity to activate displays with punch cards that print out essential facts as permanent souvenirs. The other permanent exhibit explores the cultures of the Pacific Rim countries and islands, including Japan, China, Samoa, Korea, the Philippines, New Zealand, Hawaii, and Vietnam.

Those in need of a restorative detour between the Paleozoic Era and the Ice Age might want to visit the Burke Café in the basement of the museum. It offers drinks, desserts, sandwiches, and salads in a setting reminiscent of an 18th-century music room.

➤Turn left (east) off Memorial Way onto Stevens Way. The first building on your right is the Executive Education Seminar Center. Several yards beyond is the School of Drama. At the School of Art, on the right just ahead, you can frequently watch through the ground-floor window as students work on metal art or jewelry.

➤As you wind along Stevens Way, you will note a metal framework where cadets drill with signal flags. It is next to a building devoted to military science.

➤Pause at the Gardeners' Vista on your left. From the glimpses you have here of Lake Washington and the Cascade Range, you can imagine the views students enjoy from their windows in the high-rise dormitories to your left.

➤The next building on your left is Hall Health Center and adjacent to it is the Faculty Club, which also offers terrific views of Lake Washington.

➤Continue past the Student Union Building (HUB) to the collection of buildings dedicated to the engineering sciences. Look for a sign pointing you to the Kirsten Wind Tunnel. Visitors are sometimes allowed to inspect this facility, which focuses winds of up to 200 miles an hour on truck and airplane models. The facility is a smaller-scale version of the giant wind tunnels employed by the Seattle-based Boeing Company as it designs the next generation of jetliners.

➤After visiting the wind tunnel, retrace your steps to the HUB and enter the building. It houses the UW Book Store, a large cafeteria, meeting and study rooms, an auditorium, and a full-sized bowling and billiard complex.

➤Exit the HUB at the north end, near the bookstore and bicycle shop. Follow the broad sidewalk up a series of steps and past the Henry M. Jackson School of International

Studies. To the left of the path is a secluded glade with benches and a bust of the Norwegian composer Edvard Grieg, a hint that you are approaching the Music School and the Fine Arts Quadrangle. Gothic buildings anchor the four corners of the picturesque quadrangle. Straight ahead is Denny Hall, the oldest building on campus.

➤Make a counterclockwise circuit of the quadrangle, adding a short detour, if desired, to see Denny Hall.

➤Leave the quadrangle at its southwest end and enter Red Square, which was based vaguely on the town square in Sienna, Italy. Look for the sculpture *Broken Obelisk*, by Barnett Newman, who died in 1971, one year before the work was installed here.

The most prominent building on Red Square, and on the campus, is the Suzzallo Library, built in 1926 and used by generations of students, faculty, world-renowned historians, and award-winning Northwest writers. The stunning and dead-quiet third-floor reading room resembles the interior of Canterbury Cathedral, without the altar.

The most intriguing aspects of the library's exterior are the 18 niches high in the facade of the Gothic main building. Each niche contains a sculpted figurine. The subjects were chosen in 1923 by UW faculty members from the names of 246 people nominated for their "contributions to learning and culture." No, the figure holding what appears to be a basketball is not one of the Seattle SuperSonics. It is Sir Isaac Newton, holding a globe. From left to right as you face the library entrance, the statues depict Moses, Louis Pasteur, Dante, William Shakespeare, Plato, Benjamin Franklin, Justinian, Newton, Leonardo da Vinci, Galileo, Johann Wolfgang von Goethe, Herodotus, Adam Smith, Homer, Johann Gutenberg, Ludwig van Beethoven, Charles Darwin, and Hugo Grotius. If you guessed them all, you deserve to win a 50-yard-line seat in Husky Stadium.

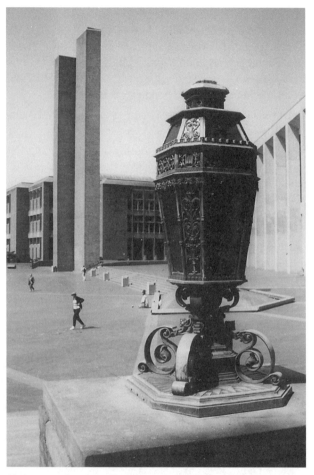

*Twin towers loom over Red Square, on the University of Washington campus. The square was designed to resemble the one in Sienna, Italy.*

On the opposite end of Red Square, past Kane Hall and the Odegaard Undergraduate Library, is a statue of George Washington commissioned by the Daughters of the American Revolution and created in 1909 by Lorado Taft. When the DAR ran short of funds, schoolchildren from around the state pitched in and contributed coins.

➤After inspecting the statue, you may want to visit the recently renovated Henry Art Gallery at this end of Red Square. The gallery features modern art, 19th-century European and American landscape paintings, photography, Indian textiles, and Northwest art. When you exit the Henry Gallery, Red Square will be on your left.

➤From the gallery, walk straight past the Allen Center for the Visual Arts.

➤Turn left back into the campus at Gate 5. This will take you past Meany Hall, on your left.

➤Bear left on Grant Lane.

➤Turn right onto the unmarked path between Johnson Hall and Mary Gates Hall. This path leads directly to Frosh Pond and Drumheller Fountain. Gates Hall was named after the mother of Microsoft founder Bill Gates. She graduated from UW in 1950 and remained an active supporter of the school until her death in 1994.

➤Go to the left around Frosh Pond. At the opposite side of the pond, look for a grove of evergreen trees. As you approach, you will note an opening in a tunnel of laurel leaves that leads to the outdoor Sylvan Theater, a hidden glade with four white columns.

➤After visiting the Sylvan Theater, return to Frosh Pond and continue your clockwise loop around it.

➤Turn left onto the path that leads between Bagley Hall and the Atmospheric Sciences Building.

➤Follow the pathway that leads diagonally to the left. This will take you to the Physics and Astronomy Building. The bowling-pin-like sculpture is *Everything That Rises*, by Martin Puryear. To your left is an observation platform that overlooks the Lake Washington Ship Canal.

➤Go down the stairway. To your left as you reach the bottom, you will see the mammoth Magnuson Health Center. But turn right onto the asphalt bike-pedestrian path, part of the Burke-Gilman Trail.

➤Cross 15th Avenue Northeast and stay on the path.

➤In one block, turn right onto University Way Northeast. On this lower portion of University, you will pass several buildings that were built or converted for university use.

➤As you continue north, you will pass the College Inn Bed and Breakfast, 4000 University Way Northeast. The UW Information Center is at the intersection of University Way and Northeast Campus Parkway. Look for La Tienda, one of the best folk-art outlets in the city, at 4138 University Way.

➤For the next few blocks, you will pass countless fast-food and ethnic restaurants, sports bars, and Husky sports apparel stores, as well as the block-long University Bookstore Complex, which starts at Northeast 43rd Street. If you need any bus schedules for your travels around Seattle, chances are you will find what you need just inside the main entrance of the bookstore.

➤Continue up University Way to Northeast 50th Street. The big yellow building at this intersection was once a school and is now University Heights Community Center.

➤Turn right and go 3 blocks to reach 17th Avenue Northeast.

➤Turn right again and head down this beautiful, broad, tree-lined boulevard, which passes through the heart of the fraternity and sorority district and leads you back to the campus entrance at Northeast 45th Street and the Burke Museum parking lot.

*walk* 15

# Washington Park Arboretum

**General location:** About 5 miles north of the city center in the Montlake District, which adjoins the University of Washington campus and Lake Washington.

**Special attractions:** A waterfront trail over Marsh and Foster Islands, arboretum, Japanese Garden, and Museum of History and Industry.

**Difficulty rating:** Moderate; there is no elevation gain, but much of the walk is over cedar-bark trails or grass.

**Distance:** 3 miles.

**Estimated time:** 1.5 hours.

**Services:** Restrooms, bookstores, and gift shops at both the Museum of History and Industry and at the arboretum visitor center.

# Washington Park Arboretum

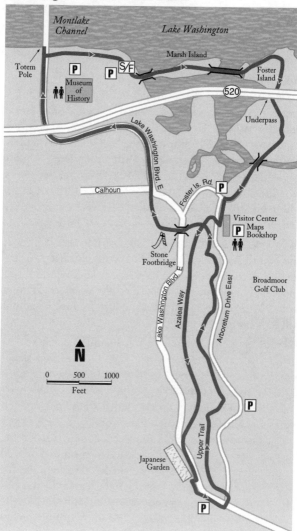

**Restrictions:** Wear stout shoes, because some paths can be muddy. No jogging is permitted on the paths. Please obey the leash and scoop laws for pets.

**For more information:** Contact the Museum of History and Industry or the Washington Park Arboretum.

**Getting started:** From downtown Seattle, drive north on Interstate 5 and take the Washington Highway 520 (Bellevue) exit. After a quarter-mile, take the Montlake Boulevard exit, also marked "University of Washington." Stay in the right lane. Go straight through the traffic light and follow the sign that says "Washington Park Arboretum." Almost immediately after crossing the intersection, you will see a sign directing you to "Historical Museum." Turn left there. The road will take you around the museum and slightly downhill to a large lot where you may park for free.

**Public transportation:** From the intersection of Pike Street and Fourth Avenue in downtown Seattle, take Metro Transit Bus 43 to the intersection of Montlake Boulevard East and East Hamlin Street. Walk three blocks east on Hamlin to the Museum of History and Industry. Husky Stadium will be on your left.

**Overview:** The Washington Park Arboretum means a lot of things to a lot of different people. Thousands of Seattle residents consider it their personal flower garden. In the springtime, lots of University of Washington students grab a book and a tree and adopt it as a secluded study hall. It is an outdoor studio for artists and nature photographers. It features a favorite fishing hole and a canoe route through the lily pads. Dates of the annual plant and bulb sales are marked on gardeners' calendars. It is everybody's favorite walk.

You would never guess that this bucolic treasure was also once the site of seething controversy, but it was. "Ban the Evergreen Bridge" rallies were staged in the arboretum before a second floating bridge across Lake Washington—now the Evergreen Point Floating Bridge—was built in 1963. A few years later, 275 members of the skinny-dipping lobby petitioned unsuccessfully to have the duck lagoon declared a nude beach.

But the arboretum also has had its staunch defenders, including Dr. Hugo Winkenwerden, a former dean of the University of Washington Forestry Department.

The roots of the arboretum extend back to 1924, when a group of Seattle gardening enthusiasts convinced city park commissioners that Seattle's climate and soil could support 98 percent of the world's plants. Ten years later, the university agreed to sponsor an arboretum project at Washington Park. The conversion of the grounds was eventually completed by the federal government during the Depression years.

Eleanor Roosevelt was once invited to the arboretum to plant a tree right next to the George Washington Elm. Originally a slip from the tree under which Washington took command of the Continental Army, the George Washington Elm was donated to the arboretum by the Daughters of the American Revolution.

Some consider the arboretum to be the university's private park, but it is operated jointly by UW and the City of Seattle. And it is not private. In fact, the support group for this 200-acre preserve numbers 3,000 members. They stage fundraising events, including sales of surplus plants, and they staff an information booth providing brochures designed to help visitors get maximum enjoyment out of a day or an hour spent roaming the paths and byways.

The arboretum now showcases 5,500 plant species suitable for the Puget Sound climate. Spring brings out the flowering cherries, azaleas, and rhododendrons. There are camellias, magnolias, and dogwoods to provide bursts of brightness through the summer. Fall brings out the leaf peepers, lured by the birches, hazels, and mountain ash among the oaks, maples, and firs. Holly trees provide bursts of winter color.

Be sure to visit the Japanese Garden, located at the opposite end of the arboretum from the visitor center. It is usually an oasis of quiet beauty. On special occasions, members of Seattle's Japanese community may offer demonstrations of drumming, storytelling, martial arts, the tea ceremony, origami, and koi fish feeding.

This walking tour begins and ends at the Museum of History and Industry, where permanent displays give visitors accurate and colorful glimpses of Seattle as it existed before, after, and during the Great Fire of 1889. There is a Boeing mail plane from the 1920s, antique cars, trolleys, and racing boats. There is even a World War II submarine with its periscope aimed at the "fleet" of cars crossing Lake Washington on the Evergreen Point Floating Bridge. The museum is open from 11 A.M. to 5 P.M. Tuesdays through Fridays and from 10 A.M. to 5 P.M. Saturdays and Sundays.

# the walk

➤Walk to the far end of the parking lot, toward Lake Washington. A path leads down to a roofed signboard. Proceed to the right on a lakeside trail that almost immediately leads you onto floating walkways that cross a marsh. The water depth next to the shore is about 6 feet, and below that are peat deposits up to 70 feet deep. Look for mallards, Canada geese, coots, grebes, bitterns, green herons, and a variety of smaller birds like song sparrows, goldfinches, and bushtits.

To your left across Union Bay is Husky Stadium. You can also see the UW boathouse, where you can rent canoes and sailboats. This bay is also the home of UW rowing crews, who are often seen working out.

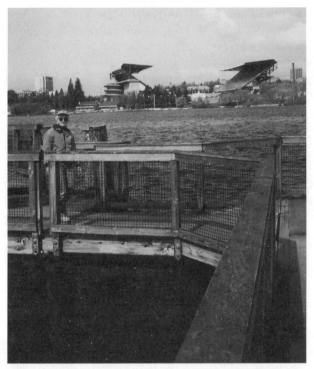

*Husky Stadium provides a visually unusual backdrop for one of the floating walkways on Lake Washington.*

Several short, bark-covered trails lead from the main pathway to spots where anglers, picnickers, photographers, and bird watchers take up station.

➤A footbridge leads you onto Foster Island. Take the path that curves right toward a pedestrian tunnel. This leads under the highway approach to the Evergreen Point Floating Bridge. You will pass a stand of maples, red cedars, madronas, and birches.

➤A small bridge leads off Foster Island. On your right is another small bay. To your left is Broadmoor, an exclusive and somewhat historic country club and gated community. As you pass the gate to Broadmoor, you will see ahead of you the first of the buildings that make up the arboretum headquarters.

➤Pass by the arboretum work yard.

➤At Arboretum Drive East, turn left and go uphill to the visitor center, which is open daily. Pick up a free trail map, browse the bookstore, and consider a restroom stop before you head out the front door and cross Arboretum Drive East into the arboretum.

➤Follow the sign leading to Azalea Way, which is particularly spectacular in the spring when the Japanese cherry trees are in bloom. Follow Azalea Way, a grass pathway, across the length of the arboretum to its end at a crosswalk over Lake Washington Boulevard East.

➤Cross the boulevard with care, turn left, and walk along the fence line to the entrance of the Japanese Garden, an oasis of tranquility with arching stone bridges, miniature waterfalls, and a stand that is used in late summer for ceremonies to celebrate the rise of the moon. There are pools filled with the colorful Japanese carp called koi, frogs among the water lilies, an occasional blue heron, a tearoom, and a 200-year-old Kobi Lantern.

➤When you exit the Japanese Garden, walk to the far end of the parking lot.

➤Carefully cross Lake Washington Boulevard and go uphill on Arboretum Drive East.

➤Almost immediately you will take a path to the left off the road. This is the start of the arboretum's Upper Trail, and it will lead you past several secluded ponds and stone

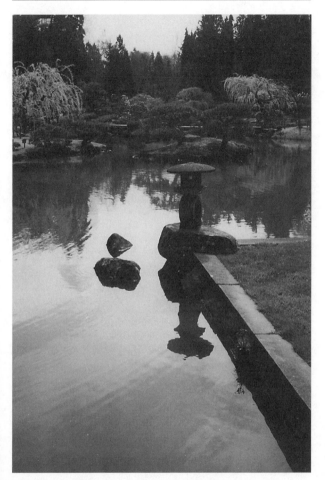

*The Japanese Garden is a tranquil oasis in the Washington Park Arboretum.*

gazebos. It is a winding trail with side spurs, but just remember to stay below the paved road as you walk back toward the visitor center.

➤Across Arboretum Drive East from the visitor center is a large, wooden map of the area. Go straight past the sign, across Azalea Way, to a stone footbridge over Lake Washington Boulevard.

➤Cross the bridge and walk through the small playground.

➤Immediately turn right onto an unmarked street, which is 26th Avenue East.

➤Walk one block, to the intersection of 26th and Calhoun Avenue, where two traffic signs read "Do Not Enter." This does not apply to pedestrians.

➤Cross Calhoun to the sidewalk and head toward Husky Stadium. This sidewalk will eventually turn left and lead you back to the entrance to the Museum of History and Industry.

➤Turn right onto the museum road, but instead of walking back to your car immediately, continue straight ahead toward the Montlake Canal. At the water's edge is a giant totem pole and wooden deck. To your left, you will see the gatekeeper's tower above the Montlake Bridge. The canal in front of you is a popular viewing area for the nautical parade saluting opening day of the Seattle pleasure boating season in the spring. Rowing crews also engage in sprint races up the canal. The slogans of some of the competing classes and schools are painted on the concrete sides of the canal.

➤Turn around and retrace your steps until you see the path leading left along the canal. Follow it to the signboard that marked the start of this walk.

### A Nautical Parade

It could be argued that every day of the year—rain or sunshine, January or July—there is a nautical parade in Seattle. You can spot the spectators in slickers or shorts, standing on the paths along Montlake Canal or strolling along the adjoining Arboretum Waterfront Trail. They might be gawking at canoeists or kayakers paddling between the University of Washington Boathouse and the various channels off Portage Bay. They might be watching a giant paddlewheel dredge, steaming between Lake Union and Lake Washington. They might be following the course of low-flying seaplanes, as they glide toward a landing. Or they might be observing national championship Husky rowing crews, stroking the calm or stormy waters during early morning workouts before their first class at the University of Washington.

Want a parade? Check Portage Bay before and after any football game played in 72,500-seat Husky Stadium. The floating tailgate parties begin just after dawn and can last long after the air horns have tooted their last supportive blasts for the UW Huskies. Restaurants on the Seattle waterfront, in Bellevue and Kirkland, and at Fisherman's Terminal in Ballard feed the fans and then transport them to the game in party-time excursion boats.

But the biggest boating parade of the year in Seattle is the opening-day boat parade, usually staged the first Saturday in May.

Again, the best viewing points are along the Montlake Canal. The day usually begins with crew races through the cut. And then the gaily decorated boating fleet sets sail through the passageway between Lake Washington and Lake Union.

Many of the participants moor their boats on the log booms a day before the event and then party into the evening. The next morning, the scent of frying bacon drifts through the mists around Foster Island.

When the cannon booms, the bands strike up, and the boat parade begins. Spectators can expect to see luxury yachts cruising through the canal, along with fireboats, tugboats, buoy tenders, and Coast Guard cutters. The number of crafts participating—decorated or undecorated—numbers upwards of 1,000.

*walk* 16

# Mercer Slough Nature Park

  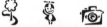

**General location:** In Bellevue, east of Lake Washington and just off Interstate 90.

**Special attractions:** Nature trails, blueberry farm.

**Difficulty rating:** Easy; flat terrain, bark paths and boardwalks. In wet weather, boots are recommended.

**Distance:** 2 miles.

**Estimated time:** 1 hour.

**Services:** Maps and other information are available at Winters House. There are restrooms and drinking fountains at Winters House and Overlake Blueberry Farm. Nature walks are conducted on Sundays and canoe trips on Saturdays. Canoe and kayak rentals are located nearby.

## Mercer Slough Nature Park

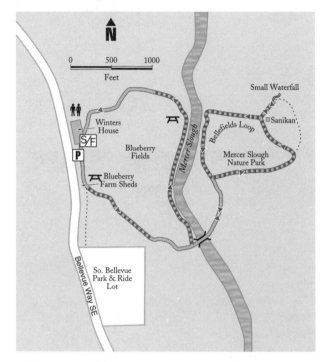

**Restrictions:** Dogs must be kept on leashes. Owners must pick up after their pets. Bicycles are allowed on exterior paved trails only. No motorized boats are allowed in Mercer Slough.

**For more information:** Contact the Bellevue Parks Department, Bellevue Historical Society, or Winters House.

**Getting started:** From I-5 Southbound, take the exit to I-90 Eastbound. Cross the Lacey V. Morrow Memorial Bridge to Mercer Island, traverse the island, and then cross the East

174

Channel Bridge back to the mainland. Take the Bellevue Way exit and pass the South Bellevue Park and Ride lot and the sign for the Overlake Blueberry Farm. Look for the blue Winters House sign on the right, at 2102 Bellevue Way Southeast. There is a parking lot adjacent to Winters House.

**Public transportation:** Board Metro Transit Bus 226 at Bay D of the Convention Place, 800 Pike Street, or at University Street stations in downtown Seattle. Get off at the South Bellevue Park and Ride lot. Follow the sidewalk to the blue Winters House sign.

**Overview:** You might see a great blue heron take flight from a rookery tree. You might glimpse a river otter, beaver, or coyote. Yet, when you look up from the trail, you will see the skyscrapers of Bellevue, less than a mile away from the Mercer Slough Nature Park.

The park encompasses 320 acres of wetland, hiking and canoe trails, a working blueberry farm, and the historic Winters House Visitor Center—all on the site where there were once commercial gardens growing fruits, vegetables, and flowers for Bellevue residents.

The hiking trails pass over and along the Mercer Slough and consist of wooden walkways and bark paths.

More than 100 species of birds live in the park, which has been described as one of the most diverse ecosystems in King County. Six enhancement ponds have been created to further increase habitat in the wetlands.

The contrast with the commercial complex in downtown Bellevue is remarkable. Whaling ships once wintered in nearby Meydenbauer Bay. To reach the east side of Lake Washington, Seattle residents had to journey around the north end of the lake or board one of the small ferries running between Seattle's Leschi Park and Meydenbauer Bay. But when two floating bridges were built to span the lake,

Bellevue was transformed from a quiet village and artists' retreat into a business and shopping center that rivals Seattle, even though Bellevue's population is only a little over 100,000.

In the pioneer days, the center of social activity on the east side of Lake Washington was Bellevue's Strawberry Festival. Today, the Pacific Northwest Arts and Crafts Festival draws artists and art lovers to Bellevue from throughout the United States. A spin-off of the festival is the Bellevue Art Museum. A visit to the museum and to the Bellevue Square shopping complex is recommended before or after the Mercer Slough Nature Park walk.

To reach the downtown core from the park, continue on Bellevue Way past the Winters House. When you reach Northeast Fourth Street, look left to see Bellevue Downtown Central Park, which features a circular walking path, reflecting canal, and waterfall. Just past the park, also on the left, is Bellevue Square. Follow the signs for free parking directly off Bellevue Way.

# the walk

➤Begin the walk on the path that leads from the Winters House past the parking area. The path leads up to a sidewalk that borders Bellevue Way Southeast.

➤Turn left down the driveway to the Overlake Blueberry Farm. It is clearly marked. At the bottom of a short slope, you will pass large metal sheds. In season, this is the headquarters for blueberry sales. You can pick your own or buy some from the vendors. A few other fruits and vegetables are also sold seasonally. There are picnic tables and toilet facilities at this location.

➤Go straight past the last shed to the wooden automobile

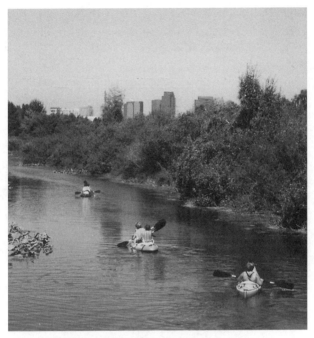

*Kayakers as well as walkers enjoy observing the wildlife and wildflowers along slow-moving Mercer Slough.*

barriers that mark the start of a pathway. Follow this bark-covered path through a green tunnel created by overhanging tree limbs.

➤When the path ends, take the boardwalk to the left. A sign points the way to "Bellefields trails." When the boardwalk curves to the left, you will be looking straight ahead at the skyscrapers in downtown Bellevue.

➤The boardwalk leads to a footbridge over the Mercer Slough. Cross the bridge. Often you will see kayakers or canoeists paddling up the serene, slow-moving slough.

➤The boardwalk continues as you leave the bridge. In late summer, the blackberry bushes on both sides of the trail invite you to participate in an instant lunch.

➤Turn right when the trail dead-ends at a T junction. A sign indicates that you are on the Bellefields Loop. The boardwalk ends and the path is now covered with bark. It passes through an area of mowed grass, tall bushes, and trees. This was once the site of pioneer homes.

➤The trail curves right. You are now in the Mercer Slough Nature Park. An interpretive sign invites you to seek out and identify footprints on the often-muddy ground beside the trail. These may have been left by coyotes, minks, raccoons, otters, or dogs. Some of the most common native plants in this area are snowberry, lady fern, Indian plum, and hazelnut. Listen for song sparrows in the willow trees.

Rivulets of water frequently cross the path. Wooden bridges, five feet in length, enable you to keep your feet dry.

A park sign informs you that if you had stood on this trail before 1917, you would have been standing on the shore of Lake Washington. The water receded 9 feet after the completion of the Lake Washington Ship Canal, which links the lake with the saltwater of Puget Sound.

There is a portable toilet next to the trail. Just past it, you will see another blue trail sign that advises you to turn left to complete the loop back toward the main bridge over the slough. Before you follow those instructions, walk 20 or 30 yards to the right from the trail sign for a glimpse of some small but picturesque waterfalls.

➤Retrace your steps to the trail sign and head left over a small bridge and back onto a bark path.

➤Ignore the wooden stairs that climb away from the path to the right. Instead, continue on the path that curves left into an area with an abundance of skunk cabbage. This area of the walk contains the ferns and other plants found in the rain forests of Washington's Olympic Peninsula.

➤Stay to the left when the bark path branches. This section of the trail is usually damp or muddy, depending upon the season.

➤When the path reaches the bank of the slough, there is a bench and another informative sign helping you identify the ducks, geese, herons, and other wetland birds you might spot from this or other viewpoints along the walk. In the autumn, you might also see spawning salmon in the slough.

➤The path continues to meander alongside the slough. Turn right at the interpretive sign that points you toward another boardwalk and the bridge over the slough.

➤Cross the bridge.

➤Turn right at the sign pointing toward the Heritage Trail and visitor center. You are now on a bark path that leads between the slough and the blueberry farm. Water lilies can frequently be seen in this stretch of the slough. A picnic table is located at the far end of the blueberry field. This vantage point offers a good view back down the slough, to the bridge and beyond.

➤Follow the path as it turns left and follows a fence line.

➤You will cross a boardwalk over an area of cattails and other marsh plants. The bright orange berries of mountain ash trees can be seen in the summer and fall. In spring, you will pass the spectacular blooms of rhododendrons, which were commercially grown at this end of the slough before the area was converted to parkland.

➤Turn right at the sign pointing you back toward the Winters House and the parking lot.

## The Winters House

The architecture seems more typical of San Diego, San Antonio, or Sonora, but the Winters House has been a part of Bellevue history since the 1920s. It is now the only structure in the city on the National Register of Historic Places.

Historians trace the Spanish influence on the house's design to a trip Frederick and Cecelia Winters took to Cuba. About the same time, Spanish Eclectic architecture, which emphasized stucco exterior walls and the generous use of colorful tiles, was enjoying great favor in California, in part due to the Panama-California Exposition held in San Diego in 1915.

The Winters House has been extensively renovated and now serves as a cultural and natural interpretive center and the home of the Bellevue Historical Society. The walls are lined with books and photographs relating to the house and to the community that surrounds it. Volunteers and staff members will provide guided tours of the house and grounds upon request.

Frederick Winters arrived in Washington from New York in 1906. After his marriage to Cecelia Roedel, the two opened a highly successful wholesale floral business. The nursery was located within the Mercer Slough watershed. The Winterses specialized in azaleas, daffodils, and irises. The house was built so that the rear windows looked out on the bulb fields and natural wetlands.

The Winterses moved from Bellevue to Vashon Island in 1943. The house and nursery were purchased by Austrian immigrants Anna and Frank Riepel. Part of the property was sold to Endre Ostbo, who opened his own rhododendron nursery as the self-proclaimed "King of the Shrubs."

The City of Bellevue purchased the former Winters estate in 1988. The well-tended grounds feature some of the nursery plants introduced by the original owners.

*walk* 17

# Kirkland

    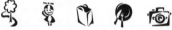

**General location:** Across Lake Washington from Seattle via Evergreen Point Floating Bridge.

**Special attractions:** Waterfront views, shops, antique stores, several restaurants.

**Difficulty rating:** Easy; flat, on sidewalks and paths, two flights of stairs.

**Distance:** 3.5 miles.

**Estimated time:** 2 hours.

**Services:** Several restaurants; restrooms and drinking fountains at Kirkland Marina Park, Marsh Park, Houghton Beach Park, and Carillon Point.

**Restrictions:** Dogs are not allowed on public beaches. Leash and scoop laws for pets are enforced.

# Kirkland

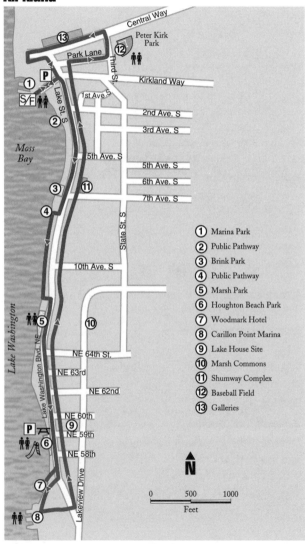

1. Marina Park
2. Public Pathway
3. Brink Park
4. Public Pathway
5. Marsh Park
6. Houghton Beach Park
7. Woodmark Hotel
8. Carillon Point Marina
9. Lake House Site
10. Marsh Commons
11. Shumway Complex
12. Baseball Field
13. Galleries

**For more information:** Contact the Kirkland Parks Department or the Kirkland Chamber of Commerce.

**Getting started:** Drive north on Interstate 5 from the Seattle city center. Exit right onto Washington Highway 520 and cross the Evergreen Point Floating Bridge. Take the Kirkland exit after crossing the bridge. Via a cloverleaf, this will direct you north onto Lake Washington Boulevard Northeast. Stay left at a Y junction and take Lake Street South. Turn left off Lake Street at Kirkland Way and proceed to Marina Park. There is free parking at the marina, with a two-hour limit.

**Public transportation:** Board northbound Metro Transit Bus 251 on Fourth Avenue in downtown Seattle. Exit at Lake Street and Kirkland Way in downtown Kirkland. Walk one block toward Lake Washington to Marina Park.

**Overview:** In 1946, just about the most exciting events to transpire in the community of Kirkland were the pig swimming contests held on Moss Bay. They were such a novelty that they were even broadcast on national radio. Identification of the porkers was a problem for the play-by-play radio announcer, who did not return for the second annual event.

Kirkland's image has changed, from rural to rich. The transition was marked in 1988 by a State Supreme Court ruling that a 13-acre Kirkland pig farm constituted a public nuisance. Today, Kirkland is one of the most affluent and sophisticated communities in the greater Seattle area. It is the home of more than a dozen art galleries and some 20 pieces of public art, ranging from the bronze *Leap Frog* sculpture by Prince Monyo Mihailescu-Nasturel to the Native American sculpture *The Water Bearers,* by Glenna Goodacre.

This walk offers glimpses of the luxurious homes and condominiums overlooking Lake Washington, passes through a series of people-friendly lakeside parks, and explores the

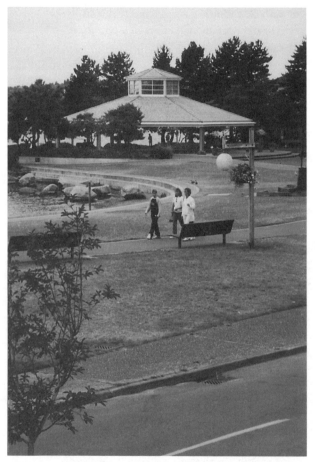

*The site of Marina Park in Kirkland was under water until 1916, when the creation of a ship canal caused the water level in the lake to drop by 9 feet.*

art and restaurant scene of this rapidly growing community surrounding Marina Park.

Marina Park did not exist until 1916, when the creation of the Lake Washington Ship Canal lowered the water level in the lake by 9 feet. The City of Kirkland eventually purchased the swampy waterfront plot that was exposed from King County for $400. Then the city created a public beach and a dock for pedestrian-only ferry service across the lake to Seattle.

Kirkland was searching for an identity almost from the time industrialist Peter Kirk arrived in the late 1880s and predicted that the area could become a steel town, a "Pittsburgh of the West." That hope died during the economic depression of 1893. For a long time after that, Kirkland was a blue-collar community dependent on the logging and transportation industries.

In recent years, communities east of Lake Washington have boomed beyond Peter Kirk's most optimistic dreams. The economic revival was not due to the "hardware" manufactured by steel mills but to the "software" created by the computer industry that attracts many of Kirkland's residents, patrons of the arts, and devotees of the active life.

Kirkland has more than 2 miles of shoreline parks, and the community recently built a new library and performing arts center. The center of activity is Lake Street South, from the downtown gallery district south along the lake to the Carillon Point complex, which includes more restaurants, more works of art, a yacht moorage, and a luxury hotel.

Lake Street is where most Kirkland residents get their exercise. Walkers, joggers, skaters, and parents pushing strollers share the sidewalk. In the summer, they pass beaches populated by sunbathers, swimmers, windsurfers, and volleyball enthusiasts.

of interest

### The Gates Mansion

Bill Gates goes to work in Redmond and lives in Medina, but it is difficult to catch a glimpse of him at either location. A lot of Seattle visitors seek out the next best option. They board a boat in Kirkland to get a look at Gates's $53 million residence.

Argosy Cruises offers aquatic tours of Lake Washington from the Kirkland waterfront. Some people take one of the 90-minute cruises to get a close-up look at the Evergreen Point Floating Bridge. Others want a glimpse of the University of Washington campus and Husky Stadium. Virtually everybody wants to see the Gates mansion in Medina.

The curious have been frustrated by Gates's desire for privacy. You cannot see his new home from the street. Only friends and personal guests get inside the Gates's gates. But you can view the terraced estate from the deck of the tour boat.

What visitors see is more than a mansion. It is less than some castles. What Gates and his architects aimed for was an electronic Shangri-La that looks more like a cluster of cabins in the woods.

Some cabins! An underground garage has space for 30 cars. A series of terraced pavilions is linked by underground passages. The reception hall can accommodate 120 guests, and the walls are lined with two dozen 40-inch television screens. When Vice President Al Gore and 100 business leaders were invited to dinner in the great hall, the Vienna Philharmonic performed during the feast.

The Gates complex includes a 60-foot indoor swimming pool, a movie theater, an 18-hole miniature golf course, and a trout stream. When a guest returns for a second visit, computers will have determined his taste in music, artwork,

**186**

lighting, and climate. An electronic pin, worn by the guest as he moves from room to room, will then adjust all these factors to the guest's satisfaction.

In 1990, when the Microsoft founder ordered construction to begin on five acres of land in Medina, Gates's net worth was estimated at $2.5 billion. When the residence was completed, in 1997, his worth had risen to $40 billion.

Financial experts predict that Gates will be able to make the payments on his "cabin in the woods."

Vehicular traffic along Lake Street is also congested. But Kirkland boosters say there is really no reason for residents to drive once they have reached their homes or apartments, many of which are on Lake Street. Almost everything they need is within walking distance. That is the concept city planners have emphasized as they encourage multifamily housing in this scenic corridor. The area has recently been called King County's Gold Coast and compared to Sausalito, the city across the bay from San Francisco.

Sausalito may be able to boast a population of seals—but Kirkland once had swimming pigs.

# the walk

➤From Marina Park, head up Kirkland Way away from Lake Washington.

➤Turn right onto Lake Street South. The business establishments you initially encounter set the tone for this youthful, energetic community. There is a bustling real estate office, an outdoor sports shop and Café Da Vinci. The latter is a sports bar, pizza parlor, and community center.

➤Just past the intersection of Lake Street South and Second Avenue South, look for a marker that reads "Public pathway, open to pedestrians 10 A.M. to dusk. Stay on path." This pathway and others like it are a compromise between property owners and the city managers, who want to make the waterfront accessible and attractive to residents and visitors.

➤Turn right onto the path and make a short detour down to Lake Washington, where there are benches and a viewpoint overlooking the colorful Kirkland marina with its pleasure craft, fireboats, and occasional government research vessels.

➤Return back up the path, turn right, and continue your walk up Lake Street. On your right is one of the impressive and expensive condominiums that have mushroomed along this main thoroughfare.

The first of the lakeside parks you pass on this walk is David E. Brink Park, which features a Native American sculpture entitled *The Water Bearers*. It was created by Glenna Goodacre in 1985. This is one of several bronze castings on display in Kirkland that is on loan from the collection of William C. Ballantine. There is a lighted dock and drinking fountain at Brink Park.

➤Turn right onto the public pathway at 733 Lake Street, just past the Lakeside condominiums. The pathway, which extends for more than 100 yards along the shore, offers a dramatic perspective of the downtown Seattle skyline. This view—comparable to ones of San Francisco—suggests why Kirkland is sometimes referred to as the Sausalito of the Northwest. The path passes a couple of mini-marinas.

➤Follow the public pathway along the shore and cross a small, wooden bridge over a tiny creek.

➤Turn left onto the path you see just before reaching Waterford East, a four-level luxury condo complex on the lakeshore.

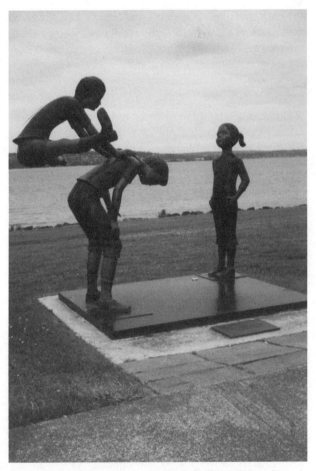

*Public art, especially sculpture, abounds in Kirkland. This sculpture in Marsh Park, called Leap Frog, was created in 1991.*

➤Return to Lake Street South and turn right. Lake Street now becomes Lake Washington Boulevard Northeast. The sidewalk takes you past Marsh Park, which also offers lakeside access, drinking fountains, and restrooms. Look for the *Leap Frog* sculpture of children at play, a bronze created by Monyo Mihailescu-Nasturel in 1991.

➤Pass to the left of Houghton Beach Park, with its children's play area, dock, drinking fountain, and restrooms. Look for another Mihailescu-Nasturel sculpture of three children. It is called *First Romance*.

A mansion identified by a sign as One Carillon Point marks the start of a complex combining a luxury hotel, office buildings, shops, restaurants, and a large marina.

➤A short way beyond the mansion, look for the marked pedestrian path to your right into Carillon Point. On a lighted pathway, you will descend a few stairs and pass through a garden of stone, wood, and metal sculptures.

➤Cross the small bridge over Carillon Creek and pass the metal sculpture of coho salmon. A salmon-rearing project is under way at this point on the creek.

➤On your left as you continue along the path is the restaurant patio of the Woodmark Hotel. Paul McCartney once stayed here. Like other guests, the former Beatle was invited to fix his own midnight snacks in the hotel kitchen.

The Carillon Point Marina, a haven for luxury yachts, is marked by two, 15-foot-tall metal structures designed to look like deep-sea fishing rods, complete with reels.

➤Walk up the double stairway leading away from the marina. At the top are gold-topped carillon towers, each of which encloses a bell that chimes on the hour. At this level, there are clothing and specialty shops, the main entrance to the Woodmark, entrances to the business towers, and underground parking.

➤Walk straight ahead past the bell towers to the traffic light.

➤Cross Lake Washington Boulevard Northeast with the light and turn left onto the sidewalk. You will now be heading back toward downtown Kirkland, but on the opposite side of the boulevard.

Across from Houghton Beach Park, note the popular sculpture of *The Story Teller,* which features three old cronies on a park bench. It is the work of R. S. Beyer and depicts "the eternal human exchange of imagination experiences."

Behind the sculpture are storyboards explaining the historical significance of the Lake House, which operated as a hotel at this site beginning in 1887. The hotel was accessible by ferry across Lake Washington and by stagecoach between Houghton and North Bend. When the railroads arrived, there was no longer much need for overnight accommodations at this particular location. But the main Lake House structure remained here until 1984.

➤Farther down Lake Washington Boulevard, past Northeast 64th Street, you will pass Marsh Commons, which features Olde English architecture. The newest residences in this mini-community of mansions sold for $800,000 and up.

➤Just past Seventh Avenue South, note on your right the Shumway complex. The tan and maroon condos are fronted by a stream, a waterfall, and a Native American sculpture. In the 1870s, Edwin and Phoebe Shumway built a mansion here on a 160-acre homestead. Their daughter became Kirkland's first city councilwoman in 1911, the same year that women were granted the right to vote in local elections. In 1982, the Shumway mansion was hauled by truck from this prime real estate and relocated in Juanita, where it reopened as reception center and a bed-and-breakfast inn.

The owners of the condos at 6736 Lake Washington Boulevard Northeast take particular pride in the floral displays on their decks, which are to your right as you continue along the boulevard.

➤Turn right onto Park Lane and enter an area of art galleries, framing shops, and antique stores. Howard/Mandville is one of the principal galleries on the lane.

If you continued straight ahead into Peter Kirk Park, you would pass the Kirkland Library; a performing arts center; and an attractive shopping, restaurant, and theater complex called Park Place.

➤But our route goes left onto Third Street. On your right, across the street, is Kirkland's baseball field.

➤Cross Central Way at the traffic light and turn left onto the sidewalk. Across the street at Second and Central, note what looks like a railroad station. This is actually a large model train and hobby shop, complete with an oversized, outdoor railway signal. On your right note Bistro Provencal, one of the most enduring French restaurants in the Puget Sound area.

➤You now enter a row of upscale art galleries, furniture stores, and interior-design specialists. Foster/White is the largest and most prestigious of the galleries.

The sculpture *Cow and the Coyote,* which you will pass, was once a landmark in Seattle's Pioneer Square. Its owner, William Ballantine, relocated it to Kirkland in 1995.

➤Use the marked crosswalk to cross Central Avenue to the Kirkland Lake Building.

➤Turn left onto the sidewalk and pass the Kirkland Roaster and Ale House. You will pass a bronze sculpture by Dan Ostermiller entitled *Close Quarters*. It features a couple of rabbits reminiscent of the one in *Alice in Wonderland*.

➤Turn right onto Lake Street South at the Triple J Cafe, passing the Lakeshore Gallery, specialty shops, and restaurants.

➤Turn right onto Kirkland Way and return to Marina Park.

*walk* 18

# Bainbridge Ferry

 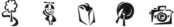

**General location:** A 35-minute ferryboat ride across Puget Sound, with portions of the walk in downtown Seattle and on Bainbridge Island.

**Special attractions:** Ferryboats, island community, waterfront park, several restaurants.

**Difficulty rating:** Easy; flat terrain except for pedestrian ramps on and off the ferryboat. Longer walk includes one uphill stint on city streets.

**Distance:** 1.5 miles if you start from the Washington State Ferry Terminal at Pier 52 on the Seattle waterfront; 3 miles if you start from Westlake Center in downtown Seattle.

**Estimated time:** The ferryboat crossing from Seattle to Winslow, on Bainbridge Island, takes 35 minutes. Because of the interval between ferry departures, you will spend a minimum

# Bainbridge Ferry (Seattle end)

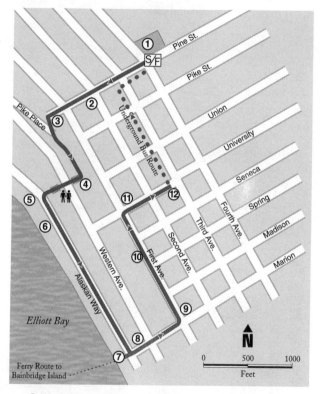

① Westlake Center
② Green Tortoise Hostel
③ Coffe Cup Sign
④ Pike St. Hillclimb & Elevator
⑤ Seattle Aquarium
⑥ Waterfront Park

⑦ Pier 52, Washington State Ferry Terminal
⑧ Overpass
⑨ Federal Building
⑩ Watermark Tower
⑪ Hammering Man
⑫ Benaroya Hall & Bus Tunnel

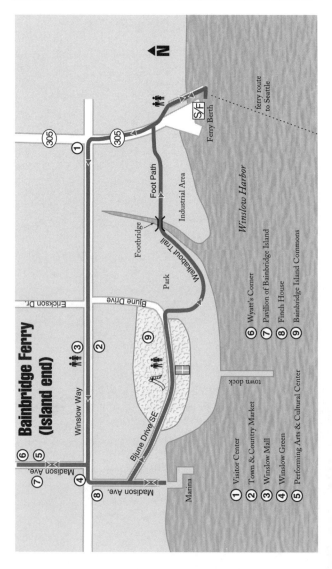

**Bainbridge Ferry (Island end)**

① Visitor Center
② Town & Country Market
③ Winslow Mall
④ Winslow Green
⑤ Performing Arts & Cultural Center
⑥ Wyatt's Corner
⑦ Pavilion of Bainbridge Island
⑧ Finch House
⑨ Bainbridge Island Commons

Winslow Harbor

ferry route to Seattle

of one hour walking and exploring Winslow. If you want to indulge in a sit-down lunch, plan on taking the second ferry, which will depart two hours after you arrive in Winslow.

**Services:** Restrooms at the ferry terminals, several restaurants, and food and restrooms on the ferryboats. Information centers at the Washington State Ferry Terminal and on Winslow Way.

**Restrictions:** With the exception of seeing-eye dogs, pets are not allowed in the ferry terminals or above deck on any ferry unless confined in a pet carrier. Walk-on passengers with pets not in carriers must board with vehicular traffic and remain on the vehicle deck. Pets must be leashed. Smoking is prohibited on the vehicle deck and in all interior spaces of the ferryboats.

**For more information:** Contact the Washington State Ferries or Team Winslow.

**Getting started:** If starting in downtown Seattle, begin at Westlake Center, at Fourth Avenue and Pine Street. If starting at the ferry terminal, it is located at Pier 52, 801 Alaskan Way. From midtown, Madison Avenue offers a direct route to the waterfront.

**Public transportation:** Downtown Seattle is a fare-free zone. Board any bus traveling south on Second Avenue. Get off at Madison Avenue and walk 3 blocks downhill to the ferry terminal.

**Overview:** When Bainbridge Island residents brag that they "walk to work" in the morning, chances are they are getting a little help from the Washington State Ferries. This walk duplicates the lifestyle of the island commuters, since it includes a ferryboat ride from Seattle to Bainbridge Island and back.

How far you walk depends upon how many laps of the

sun deck you can complete aboard one of the big ferries, which are capable of carrying more than 200 cars, trucks, and buses and more than 2,000 passengers. The largest ferries measure 460 feet in length, which means that, on the average boat, about six laps would equal a mile.

The destination on this 35-minute cruise is the tourist-friendly community of Winslow. At least it used to be known by that name. In an effort to better manage growth in the area, all of Bainbridge Island was incorporated as a "city" in 1991. The island now has some 20,000 residents, and a fourth of them reside in what was formerly the city of Winslow.

The lure of island living and a ferryboat commute are reflected in these statistics:

- Some 100 authors live on Bainbridge Island, including such best-selling writers as David Guterson, Jack Olsen, and Rebecca Wells.

- Ninety percent of island residents hold library cards.

- Forty percent of island workers commute to jobs in Seattle.

- Almost half of the island's adults have college degrees, or twice the state average.

- And, to borrow a line from Garrison Keillor, "all the children are above average." Nine out of 10 high school graduates go on to college.

If that does not convince you of the caliber of people who choose to inhabit Bainbridge Island, how about this: There is a winery within walking distance of what is now referred to as "downtown Bainbridge Island." In this same area, there are four art galleries, three bookstores, some 15 restaurants, a waterfront park, boat rentals, and a cultural center.

# the walk

➤To begin the longer version of this walk, exit the Westlake Center at Fourth Avenue and Pine Street. Head west down Pine Street toward the waterfront.

Glance to your left at Second and Pine and you will see the Green Tortoise Hostel. This is an offshoot of the Green Tortoise bus service, which once carried the "flower people" from Seattle to San Francisco, making a few picnic, beach, and spa stops along the way. The Green Tortoise buses were said to be powered by "good vibrations" and to belch incense from their exhaust pipes.

The intersection of First Avenue and Pine Street is the hub of a recently developed shopping district featuring expensive women's clothing.

➤Walking on the left (south) side of Pine, you will come to a large coffee-cup sign. Turn left here and breathe in the scent of hot soup (from Sisters' European lunch spot), Mexican produce (from El Mercado Latino Foods), and spicy chicken dishes (from Copacabana Cafe). Note also on your left the Made in Washington store and the indoor market that surrounds it.

➤Continue straight ahead past the Three Girls Bakery until you come to the sign that says "Pike Street Hillclimb."

➤Turn right just past the life-sized piggy bank and go down the stairs. There are public restrooms at the bottom of the first flight, which ends at Western Avenue. The stairs wind around. Resist the impulse to venture off into the side arcades.

➤Use the crosswalk to cross Western and continue down another winding staircase, passing ice cream and coffee shops and one of the market's most popular restaurants, El Puerco Lloron.

➤Use the crosswalk to cross Alaskan Way to the Seattle Aquarium and then turn left. You will pass the fountains of Waterfront Park and a statue of Christopher Columbus. A historical marker points out the spot where, in 1897, prospectors unloaded from the *SS Portland* the famous "ton of gold" that touched off the Klondike gold rush.

➤Continue walking down Alaskan Way, along the waterfront. Yes, it is OK if you pause to make a purchase at the frankfurter stand. The kielbasa with sauerkraut and hot mustard is recommended. But do not tarry too long. You have to catch a ferry.

The ferry terminal is just past Ivar's Acres of Clams—the statue of the founder, Ivar Haglund, feeding French fries to the seagulls—and the Seattle fireboat dock and station.

## The short version of the walk begins here:

➤Turn right and take the elevator or walk up the ramp into the Washington State Ferry Terminal. The ticket booth is at the far end of the lobby. Fares are periodically adjusted, but you should pay about $3.60 per person to make the round trip to Winslow—half that for seniors or small children. There are no collections on the Winslow end of the run.

➤Follow the crowd when the gates swing open to admit passengers to the ferry. The trip across Elliott Bay to Bainbridge Island takes 35 minutes. There is a cafeteria aboard the ferry, but if you are out for the exercise, see how many laps of the sun deck you can complete before the captain signals the end of the run with a toot of his horn.

➤Get off the ferry using the overhead ramp and follow the car and passenger traffic up the hill. You will be on a sidewalk on the right side of Washington Highway 305.

➤Turn left and cross the street at the stoplight, where the sign directs you to the city center. You can pick up a map at

**of interest**

### The Ferry Fleet

And in the beginning, there were "mosquitoes." Actually, they were independently owned and operated steamers, which traveled from the Seattle waterfront to other ports along Puget Sound in the 1800s. Together, they became known as the Mosquito Fleet, because of the way the small boats seemed to flit in and out of the landings, pausing only long enough to discharge some passengers and take on others.

In 1860, the ship *Bainbridge,* owned by the Eagle Harbor Transportation Company, was the first steel-hulled vessel to make an island run, carrying passengers and supplies from Seattle to Winslow. Well over 100 small ships—capable of hauling 200 to 400 passengers plus cargo—traveled regular routes to ports small and large. At one time, Bainbridge Island alone had 20 landings. Sixty years later, most of the Mosquito Fleet had been replaced by ferries, carrying both cars and passengers from Tacoma and Vashon Island in the south to the San Juan Islands in the north.

The Washington State Ferries system now has some 30 boats, which ferry close to 20 million passengers a year. Headquarters for the ferry system is Colman Dock on Pier 52, where a historic clock is on display. The four-sided clock sat in a tower 73 feet above the Seattle waterfront until one night in 1912, when the *Alameda,* piloted by John "Dynamite" O'Brien, slammed into the dock at almost full speed, toppling the tower, and sinking a sternwheeler on the other side. The tower was discovered the next morning, floating in Elliott Bay, the clock's hands frozen at 10:23 P.M.

Eventually, the clock was installed in a new tower, but it was later removed. It was eventually rediscovered in a chicken coop at 12th Avenue and Jackson Street. In 1984, the ferry commission acquired the clock, had it repaired, and returned it a year later to a place of honor in the Washington State Ferry Terminal.

On rare occasions, because of an engine malfunction or computer glitch, the braking system on a ferry will fail and the dock will rock from the collision. But the Colman clock never misses a tick.

this intersection, at the Chamber of Commerce Visitor Center.

➤Heading into Winslow along Winslow Way, you will pass ice cream shops, antique stores, a pizza parlor, and the Town and Country Market, where you can stock up on picnic fare. In midtown, you will come to two-story Winslow Mall on the right, which has public restrooms. There are bookstores on both sides of the street.

➤At the next major intersection, Winslow Way and Madison Avenue, is Winslow Green, which features condos and a variety of food and specialty shops.

➤Take a brief detour to your right, up Madison Avenue. After a block, note the arrow on the right pointing to the Performing Arts Cultural Center and the Farmers Market. The latter is open on weekends. Stay on the right side of the street until you reach a gazebo at Wyatt's Corner. Across the street is a former farmhouse, now the Four Swallows Restaurant.

➤Cross Madison Avenue and head back toward Winslow Way. You will pass Pavilion of Bainbridge Island, a recently built multi-screen theater and retail complex. You will also pass a combination diner and car-care center and then the popular San Carlos Mexican restaurant.

➤Cross Winslow Way and head down Madison toward the

masts you will see in the marina. Use the path on the right side of the street, which passes some turn-of-the-20th-century homes—unless the explosion of condominiums in Winslow gets to that area before you do. A travel agency and bookstore in Finch House, once the Winslow Post Office operated by "Grandpa" William Finch, is worth a second look.

▶Madison ends at the Madrona Waterfront Cafe and the marina. To the right is Pegasus Coffee Shop. In 1937, it was Anderson Hardware. Wander around the picturesque marina, waterfront, and adjoining shops and then head back up Madison, retracing your steps until you reach Bjune Drive Southeast, a block before Winslow Way.

▶Turn right onto Bjune and follow the sidewalk to a park with a children's playground. Go to the right around the slide. A path heads downhill toward the tennis courts and passes the Bainbridge Island Commons.

▶Turn right where the paths intersect and pass the grandstand shaped like a boat. At the end of the park, you will see the Walkabout Trail, which leads downhill toward a wooden footbridge.

▶Follow the Walkabout Trail, which is lighted at night, until you see a sign directing you to veer left and walk uphill one block.

▶Use care crossing WA 305 at the marked crosswalk, and then follow the crowd to the ferry terminal. Walk into and through the lobby and then left up the ramp to the waiting boat.

### The short version of the walk ends here. The longer walk continues:

▶When you exit the ferry in Seattle, do not descend the stairway to the street. Instead, go straight ahead across a

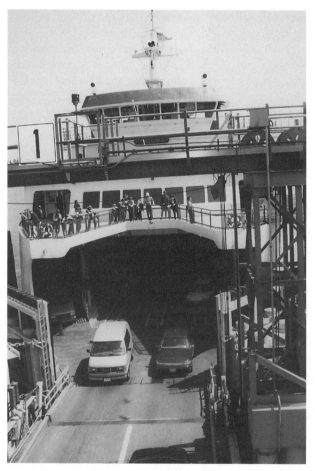

*Pedestrians await their turn as vehicles debark from the ferry Tacoma.*

pedestrian overpass. There will be auto traffic just below you and just above, on Alaskan Way. This walkway takes you to the intersection of First Avenue and Marion Street.

➤Turn left, cross to the other side of Marion, and head up First Avenue. On your right, you will pass the Federal Building and Warshall's, a longtime sporting goods store; on the left are the Alexis Hotel and Watermark Tower, one of the first high-rise condominiums erected between First Avenue and the waterfront.

➤Turn right at the *Hammering Man* sculpture at First Avenue and University Street. Go one block to the Metro tunnel station beneath the new Benaroya Hall. Any northbound bus will take you through the tunnel and back to Westlake Center, free of charge.

*walk* 19

# Sammamish River Trail

**General location:** About 12 miles north of downtown Seattle, in Bothell.

**Special attractions:** Picturesque stream, parks, Chateau Ste. Michelle and Columbia wineries, and Redhook Brewery.

**Difficulty rating:** Moderate; relatively long hike, but the trail is flat and paved.

**Distance:** 7 miles out and back. Route can be shortened to any length, but only those walking the entire distance will be able to visit the brewery and wineries.

**Estimated time:** 3.5 hours.

**Services:** Restrooms at Bothell Landing Park and at Chateau Ste. Michelle. Food services at both ends of the trail.

**Restrictions:** Pets must be leashed to avoid endangering bicyclists.

**Sammamish River Trail**

CITY OF BOTHELL

To Lake Forest Park

522

Bothell Way

N

0  0.5  1
Miles

To Kirkland

100th NE

Bothell Landing Park

Bothell Way

S/F

Footbridge

P

Brackert's Landing

To Everett, Mukilteo

405

Highway, Railroad Bridges

405

522

CITY OF WOODINVILLE

To Redmond

405

NE 143rd Place

Columbia Winery

*Sammamish River*

Woodinville - Redmond Road

Wilmot Gateway Park

Vegetable, Flower Gardens

Gold Creek Complex

S/F

Turnaround Point

NE 145th St.

Chateau Ste. Michelle Winery

Redhook Brewery

207

**For more information:** Contact the King County Parks Department, Chateau Ste. Michelle Winery, Columbia Winery, or Redhook Brewery.

**Getting started:** From central Seattle, drive north on Interstate 5. Exit onto Washington Highway 520 and cross Evergreen Point Floating Bridge. Take the I-405 Northbound exit. Continue north on I-405 and take the Bothell exit. As you enter downtown Bothell, turn left onto Northeast 180th Street. Follow the signs downhill to the river and Bothell Landing Park. Use the free parking area across the street from the park.

**Public transportation:** From any downtown Seattle bus tunnel station, catch Metro Transit Bus 307 from Bay A. Get off at Bothell Way and Northeast 180th Street. Walk two blocks back down Bothell Way to 178th Street, and look for the Bothell Landing Park signs.

**Overview:** When the Burke-Gilman Trail and the Sammamish River Trail were linked on National Trails Day—June 5, 1993—the result was a 27-mile recreation parkway running from the heart of Seattle to suburban Redmond. On sunny days, walkers, joggers, sloggers, skaters, and cyclists share the paths with young couples walking dogs or pushing strollers. Hot-air balloons often drift overhead.

This walk covers a 3.5-mile section of the Sammamish River Trail, between Bothell Landing Park and the Chateau Ste. Michelle Winery; it returns over the same route.

The late U.S. Senator Warren Magnuson first suggested building a trail on an abandoned corridor of railway right-of-way on the west shore of Lake Washington. In 1971, the Burke-Gilman Trail was created. It was named after Judge Thomas Burke and Daniel Gilman, architects of the north-south railroad line. Today, the paved trail passes through the Fremont District of Seattle, past Gasworks Park and the University of Washington campus, and along the shores of Lake Washington to suburban Kenmore.

The Burke-Gilman Trail connects with the paved Sammamish River Trail in the Kenmore-Bothell area. The latter passes farmland, recreation fields, and industrial parks on its way to Marymoor Park in Redmond, another widely used recreation site.

The Sammamish River was a slough before it was dredged to control flooding in the 1960s. Trees along the river were cut down, and the channel was deepened and straightened. The river and 14-mile trail connect Lake Sammamish with Lake Washington.

In an average year, 500,000 people use all or part of the linked trails. A 15-mile-per-hour speed limit for bicyclists is enforced.

# the walk

➤From the parking lot at Bothell Landing Park, cross the semicircular footbridge over the Sammamish River.

➤Turn left onto the paved path. A sign warns you that "It is unlawful to hit or chase chickens or waterfowl." There are some colorful chickens running wild in this area along with lots of ducks and Canada geese. Semi-permanent house trailers line the placid river.

➤Continue to follow the path as it leads you to the left across another bridge spanning the river. For the next 3 miles, the river will be on your right.

After a long block, the paved path ends but is replaced by a broad sidewalk. On your right is Brackett's Landing, a mini-park and picnic spot on the edge of the river.

➤Turn left across the unmarked road at Brackett's Landing, and use the crosswalk to reach the sidewalk.

►Turn right and walk straight ahead on the sidewalk that leads back onto the paved trail. Bicycle usage on the trail is often heavy. Redmond, at the far end of the Sammamish River Trail, is the site of a cycling velodrome. The community has played host to several national championship races. But on the trail, cyclists usually pass you on the left and inform you verbally of their intentions.

►The path goes downhill and across another small bridge over a creek feeding the Sammamish. The path then passes under a highway cloverleaf marked by a forest of giant concrete pilings. The river flows slowly between banks covered with grass and vines. This is a popular place to gather blackberries in late summer.

For the next couple of miles, the river serves as a dividing line. To your right, across the river, the land is being developed for light industry, lumberyards, warehouses, and office parks. To your left, the land use becomes increasingly agricultural. In the summer, you can glimpse vast fields of flowers, acres of vegetables and cornstalks, and plots of sunflowers. Many of the farmers are immigrants from Southeast Asia. They sell their wares at Pike Place Market in downtown Seattle and at various community street markets, where you can see girls as young as 5 or 6 learning from their mothers the art of arranging flowers and ferns into bouquets. Their produce is among the most highly prized by shoppers at Pike Place Market.

►The path crosses yet another small bridge over a small tributary and then passes under a railroad trestle and an automobile bridge that carries light traffic over the Sammamish River toward WA 202.

►The trail now passes recently developed Wilmont Gateway Park, which features covered picnic tables, restrooms, a children's playground, a canoe and raft launch, and a grassy amphitheater for summer concerts.

Just a few hundred feet farther along the trail is a path on the left. It leads to Woodin Creek Park, a Woodinville city mini-park with picnic tables and tennis courts. Woodin Creek is part of a Sammamish habitat-restoration project designed to "make the river bank a better place for fish and people," according to a sign posted outside the park. The small creek, once relegated to an underground pipe by development, has been returned to its natural state, promoting the return of cutthroat trout, which are native to the Sammamish River.

►Continue along the main trail. You will next pass an apartment complex with a private, trailside swimming pool. Much of the Sammamish River farmland is concentrated to your left, just past the apartment complex.

Past the acres of farmland on your left is the Gold Creek recreational area, a private development not directly accessible from the Sammamish River Trail. It features picnic grounds, a golf driving range, a round structure originally built for indoor ice skating, and several buildings housing indoor tennis courts and other facilities.

From this point on the trail, you can glimpse straight ahead the green, sloping roofs of the Redhook Brewery. Just before you reach the access road to the brewery and wineries, note on your left four baseball fields comprising the North Shore Little League complex. There are restrooms and drinking water just off the trail.

►Bear left at a Y junction. The right-hand path leads along the river to Redmond and the end of the Sammamish River Trail. The left spur winds right over a newly constructed footbridge. Look to the left as you cross the bridge for a

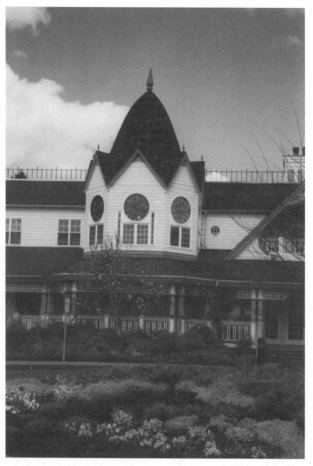

*This picturesque structure houses the tasting room of the Columbia Winery, founded in 1962 by a group made up mostly of University of Washington professors.*

good glimpse of the Sammamish Valley and fields of grass being grown commercially to make sod for "instant lawns."

The pedestrian and bicycle path, which runs parallel to Northeast 145th Street, leads directly to the Redhook brewery, offices, beer garden, and restaurant. Once a microbrewery, Redhook outgrew its former quarters in the Fremont District of Seattle. The current facility offers a limited luncheon menu and beverages served indoors at Forecasters Pub. Outdoor tables sit beside the Sammamish River.

➤Continue up the same pathway beside Northeast 145th Street to Columbia Winery, which looks like an 1880s beach pavilion. The building was actually erected within the past decade to showcase the winery, which was founded in 1962 by ten friends, seven of whom were University of Washington professors.

Inside the building, designed with a main cupola and flanking balconies, is a large tasting room with a souvenir and gift shop. The Spirit of Washington Dinner Train, which begins its daily runs in Renton, stops here so that passengers can taste the Columbia wines. It then begins its return run to Renton. Tours of the winery for the general public are available on weekends.

➤Pause before you cross Northeast 145th Street to get to Chateau Ste. Michelle. Traffic along this road can be heavy; cross with care.

➤Enter the winery gate and follow the long pathway past the rows of grapevines and into the estate, which once belonged to timber baron Fred Stimson. The white summer home of the Stimson family still sits on the grounds, surrounded by streams, ponds, fountains, and flower-lined pathways. After the property was acquired by Chateau Ste. Michelle, the other buildings were built to resemble a French country estate.

**of interest**

## Wine Country

There is a classic putdown among wine enthusiasts: After inspecting the label of an inferior selection, a wine snob will remark, "Ah, this is a good vintage: Thursday."

Until the 1960s, almost every wine produced in the state of Washington "tasted like Thursday." Fortified apple wine, in bottles that fit nicely into back pockets, probably enjoyed the greatest popularity.

True, a few grapevines were planted in the Columbia River Valley in the 1950s. Then, in 1962, some University of Washington professors founded a small winery based on their audacious assumption that classic, European-style fine wines could be produced in this area.

But it was not until 1974, when a white Riesling produced by Chateau Ste. Michelle was named "best in America" by the *Los Angeles Times*, that skepticism vanished and a new state industry was truly born.

Today, there are more than 100 wineries in the state producing award-winning Rieslings, Chardonnays, Cabernets, Merlots, Sauvignon Blancs, Syrahs, Pinot Gris, and Gewürztraminers. Most of these grapes are grown in the Yakima Valley, a two-hour drive south of Seattle. Chateau Ste. Michelle and Columbia grow their grapes in the Yakima Valley and the Columbia Basin and bottle their wine at their Sammamish Valley facilities.

In the Yakima Valley, vineyards are just part of the rural landscape, tucked among horse ranches, cornfields, and dairy farms. The main wine-growing area begins at Union, just outside Yakima, and extends to the Tri-Cities—Richland, Kennewick, and Pasco—along the Columbia River, the state's southern border.

The story of Washington wines is told during guided tours and tastings like the ones at Chateau Ste. Michelle. These are conducted seven days a week. Yup, even on Thursday.

Behind the visitor center, a vast lawn slopes downhill toward a stage. Here, summer picnic concerts feature some of the world's top recording stars. There is another picturesque picnic area on the property. It is near the vineyard and adjacent to a pond. You can buy picnic snacks and cold wines in the gift shop and enjoy them on outdoor tables.

After you have savored the life of a French grandee, head back down the Sammamish River Trail to Bothell Landing.

# Appendix A: Other Sights

There are several other popular attractions in or near Seattle. Although they may not involve walking, you may still enjoy them.

## In Seattle

**Experience Music Project:** Microsoft co-founder Paul Allen provided most of the financial backing for this rock- and pop-music hall of fame in a futuristic building on the Seattle Center grounds.

**International District:** The Wing Luke Museum, the Nippon Kan Theater, a fortune cookie company, and a 4-ton stone lantern at Kobe Terrace are among the landmarks in this Asian neighborhood, a five-minute walk from Pioneer Square. You can sample the foods of China, Japan, the Philippines, Vietnam, and Thailand in the many ethnic restaurants. The mammoth, Japanese-owned complex called Uwajimaya offers everything from quail eggs and broiled eel to Kokeshi dolls and porcelain saucers priced at a thousand dollars apiece.

**Museum of Flight:** At the heart of this aviation museum, 15 minutes from downtown Seattle, is the Red Barn, the original factory for the Boeing Company. Historic aircraft are suspended from the ceiling of this glassed-in museum. You can also explore several ground-level aerospace exhibits, as well as a simulated landing tower in which the history and development of air-traffic control are described.

**Nordic Heritage Museum:** This museum in Ballard honors all Scandinavian immigrants and traces their contributions to the Pacific Northwest. The first-floor, permanent exhibit is "Dream of America: The Immigrant Experience 1840-1920." On the second floor, exhibits focus on the fishing and logging industries. You will find displays of costumes, textiles, and tools the Scandinavian immigrants brought with them from their homelands.

**Odyssey Maritime Discovery Center:** Located on the Seattle waterfront, the center contains interactive displays in three galleries. They are devoted to the themes "Sharing the Sound," "Harvesting the Sea," and "Ocean Trade." Learn how to paddle a kayak, navigate a container ship into Elliott Bay, and locate pollock with an electronic fish finder.

**Pacific Science Center:** Located in the Seattle Center just below the Space Needle, this attractive complex of arches, pools, and five interconnecting buildings offers interactive displays of particular appeal to teenagers and families. Featured are fascinating virtual-reality demonstrations and adventures aboard a 22-foot "starship," confrontations in a robot world, and rides atop a "gravity bicycle." A new IMAX theater, opened in 1998, adjoins the science center. And do not miss the Tropical Butterfly House and Insect Village, illuminated by 28,000 watts of full-spectrum, artificial light.

**Seattle Aquarium:** This waterfront attraction offers a simulated walk on the ocean floor and a diver's view of sharks, octopuses, and 366 species of fish. Divers feed the fish at 1:30 P.M., the otters and seals at 11:30 A.M. and 2 and 5 P.M. The aquarium staff also sponsors whale-watching cruises from Everett and Anacortes.

## Outside Seattle
**Blake Island:** Scenic 8-mile cruises from Piers 55 and 56 on the Seattle waterfront run daily to this 475-acre marine park featuring Tillicum Village, where cedar-planked salmon dinners are served in a giant longhouse, accompanied by Indian dancing. There are nature trails on the forested island and Indian craft demonstrations.

**Boeing Company Tours:** More than 2 million visitors have toured the Boeing plant in Everett. The 70-minute program includes a video show, a drive past the flight line, and a bird's-eye view of the 747 or 777 production line from a high balcony.

**Emerald Downs:** Located midway between Seattle and Tacoma, Emerald Downs is the premier showcase for thoroughbred racing in the Pacific Northwest. Restaurants and food courts have been incorporated into the six-level grandstand facility. The racing season runs from April into September.

**Snoqualmie Falls:** Stand on a viewing platform in the spray of the 268-foot waterfall or watch the falls from a dining room at the posh Salish Lodge Resort just above the thundering cascade. Snoqualmie Falls is about 20 miles east of Seattle via Interstate 90.

**Washington State History Museum:** You could spend most of a day exploring the exhibits in this large museum overlooking Tacoma's working harbor. The realities of frontier life in the Puget Sound area, including the Klondike gold rush, labor strife, and the canning, lumber, mining, and shipbuilding industries are presented in re-creations, recordings, and early photographs, and in 50 interactive displays.

Next door to the history museum is Tacoma's **Union Station,** which underwent a $57 million transformation into a federal office building in 1991. Glasswork by internationally acclaimed artist Dale Chihuly is spectacularly displayed.

# Appendix B: Contact Information

Throughout this book, we have advised you to contact local attractions, museums, and shops to confirm opening times, locations, and entrance fees. The list below gives you the phone numbers and addresses of the places we have mentioned.

## Community Resources

**Seattle-King County Convention and Visitors Bureau,** Washington State Convention and Trade Center, 800 Convention Place, Seattle 98101; 206-461-5840.
Open 9 A.M. to 5 P.M. Mondays through Fridays during the winter, 9 A.M. to 5 P.M. daily during the summer.

**Ballard Chamber of Commerce,** 2208 Market Street NW, Seattle 98107; 206-784-9705.

**East King County Convention and Visitors Bureau,** 520 112th Avenue NE, Bellevue 98004; 425-455-1926.

**Fremont Chamber of Commerce,** P.O. Box 31139, Seattle 98103; 206-632-1500.

**City of Kirkland,** 123 Fifth Avenue, Kirkland 98033; 425-828-1111.

**Madison Park Community Council,** 206-325-0742.

**Queen Anne Chamber of Commerce,** P.O. Box 19386, Seattle 98109; 206-293-6876.

**Team Winslow,** P.O. Box 11379, Bainbridge Island 98110; 206-842-2982.

## Activities, Attractions, and Museums

**Alki Point Light Station,** 3201 Alki Avenue SW, Seattle 98116; 206-932-5800.
The lighthouse and support buildings are open to the public

for tours from noon to 4 P.M. on Saturdays, Sundays, and most holidays, from May through September.

**Argosy Cruises,** Pier 55, Suite 201, Seattle 98101; 206-623-4252.

**Bellevue Art Museum,** 301 Bellevue Square, Bellevue 98004; 425-454-3322.

**Bellevue Historical Society,** 425-450-1046.

**Boeing Company Tours,** 3003 W. Casino Road, Everett 98204; 800-464-1476.

Tickets are available at the plant on the day of the tour. Admission is $5 for adults, $3 for seniors and children under 16.

**Burke Museum,** NE 45th Street and 16th Avenue NE, University of Washington campus, Seattle, 98195; 206-543-5590.

Open from 10 A.M. to 5 P.M. daily except Thursdays, when hours are 10 A.M. to 8 P.M. Prices are $5.50 for adults, $4 for seniors, and $2.50 for children. Kids under 5 are admitted free. For another $1, you can also visit the Henry Art Gallery, also on campus.

**Chateau Ste. Michelle Winery,** 14111 NE 145th Street, Woodinville 98072; 206-488-3300.

Tastings and tours are available between 10 A.M. and 4:30 P.M. seven days a week, with the exception of Thanksgiving, Christmas, New Year's Day, and Easter.

**Columbia Winery,** 14030 NE 145th Street, Woodinville 98072; 425-488-2776.

Open Mondays from 10 A.M. to 5 P.M., Tuesdays through Sundays from 10 A.M. to 7 P.M. Tours and wine tastings offered Saturdays and Sundays from 10:30 A.M. to 4:40 P.M. and at other times by appointment.

**Frye Art Museum,** 704 Terry Avenue, Seattle 98104-2019; 206-622-9250.

Open Tuesdays, Wednesdays, Fridays, and Saturdays from 10 A.M. to 5 P.M., Thursdays from 10 A.M. to 9 P.M., and Sundays from noon to 5 P.M. No admission fee.

**Henry Art Gallery,** 15th Avenue NE and NE 41st Street, University of Washington campus, Seattle 98195; 206-543-2280.

Open Tuesdays, Fridays, Saturdays, and Sundays from 11 A.M. to 5 P.M., Wednesdays and Thursdays from 11 A.M. TO 8 P.M. Admission is $5 for adults and $3 for seniors. UW students and children admitted free.

**Hiram M. Chittenden Locks,** U.S. Army Corps of Engineers, 3015 NW 54th Street, Seattle 98107; visitor center 206-783-7059, administrative offices 206-783-7001.

The visitor center is open daily during the summer from 11 A.M. to 5 P.M. and Thursdays through Mondays the remainder of the year. Free guided tours of the locks, fish ladder, and garden begin at 2 P.M. on Saturdays and Sundays.

**Log House Museum,** 3003 61st Avenue SW, Seattle 98116; 206-938-5293.

Operated by the Southwest Seattle Historical Society, the museum is open Thursdays from noon to 6 P.M., Fridays from 10 A.M. to 3 P.M., and Sundays from noon to 3 P.M. A donation of $2 for adults and $1 for children is suggested. A gift shop is behind the museum.

**Museum of Flight,** 9494 E Marginal Way S (Boeing Field), Seattle 98108; 206-764-5720.

Open daily except Christmas and Thanksgiving. Hours are from 10 A.M. to 5 P.M. except Thursdays, when the museum is open from 10 A.M. to 9 P.M. Admission is $8 for adults, $7 for seniors, and $4 for students 5 to 17. No admission fee is charged between 5 P.M. and 9 P.M. on Thursdays.

**Museum of History and Industry,** 2700 24th Avenue E, Seattle 98112-2009; 206-324-1126; www.historymuse-nw.org.

Open Tuesdays through Fridays from 11 A.M. to 5 P.M. and Saturdays and Sundays from 10 A.M. to 5 P.M. Closed Mondays. Admission is $5.50 for adults, $3 for seniors and children ages 6 to 12, and $1 for children 2 to 5. Children under 2 admitted free.

**Nordic Heritage Museum,** 3014 NW 67th Street, Seattle 98117; 206-789-5707.

Open Tuesdays through Saturdays from 10 A.M. to 4 P.M. and Sundays from noon to 4 P.M. Admission for adults is $4, students and seniors $3, children 4 and under free.

**Odyssey Maritime Discovery Center,** 2205 Alaskan Way, Pier 66, Seattle 98121; 206-374-4000.

Summer hours are Sundays through Wednesdays from 10 A.M. to 9 P.M. and Thursdays through Saturdays from 10 A.M. to 5 P.M. Winter hours are 10 A.M. to 5 P.M. daily. Admission is $6.50 for adults and $4 for seniors, students, and children 5 and older. Children under 5 admitted free.

**Pacific Science Center,** 200 Second Avenue N, Seattle 98109; 206-443-2001.

Open weekdays from 10 A.M. to 5 P.M. and weekends from 10 A.M. to 6 P.M. Admission is $7.50 for adults, $5.50 for children 3 to 13 and seniors 65 and over.

**Redhook Brewery,** 14300 NE 145th Street, Woodinville 98072; 425-483-3232.

Brewery tours are offered Mondays through Fridays at 2 P.M., 3 P.M., and 4 P.M. and Saturdays and Sundays on the hour from noon to 5 P.M. The tour costs $1, including beer samples, and lasts about 40 minutes.

**Seattle Aquarium,** 1438 Alaskan Way, Seattle 98104; 206-386-4320.

Open from 10 A.M. to 5 P.M. daily, except during the summer, when hours are 10 A.M. to 7 P.M.

**Seattle Art Museum,** 100 University Street, Seattle 98101; 206-654-3100.

Open Tuesdays through Sundays from 10 A.M. to 5 P.M. and Thursdays from 10 A.M. to 9 P.M. Admission is $6 for adults, $4 for seniors and students.

**Seattle Asian Art Museum,** Volunteer Park, Seattle 98112; 206-654-3100.

Open Tuesdays, Wednesdays, Fridays, Saturdays, and Sundays from 10 A.M. to 5 P.M. Open Thursdays from 10 A.M. to 9 P.M. Admission is $6 for adults and $4 for students and seniors. Children under 12 admitted free.

**Space Needle,** 219 Fourth Avenue N, Seattle Center, Seattle 98109; 206-443-2111.

Elevator to observation deck operates from 8 A.M. to 11 P.M. daily. Admission $8.50 for adults, $7 for seniors, $5 for children 5 to 12.

**Tillicum Village,** 2200 Sixth Avenue S, Suite 804, Seattle 98121; 206-443-1244.

**University of Washington Visitor Center,** 4014 University Way, Seattle 98195; 206-543-9198.

Open 8 A.M. to 5 P.M. Mondays through Fridays.

**University of Washington Observatory,** NE 45th Street and 17th Avenue NE, Seattle 98195; 206-543-0126.

Open to the public most Mondays and Thursdays.

**Windsor Olson Crime Tours,** 2450 Sixth Avenue S, Suite 1A, Seattle 98134; 206-622-0590.

**Wing Luke Asian Museum,** 407 Seventh Avenue S, Seattle 98104; 206-623-5124.

Open Tuesdays through Fridays from 11 A.M. to 4:30 P.M. and weekends from noon to 4 P.M. Admission is $2.50 for adults, $1.50 for students and seniors, and 75 cents for children 5 to 12. Admission is free on Thursdays.

**Woodland Park Zoo,** 5500 Phinney Avenue N, Seattle 98103; 206-684-4800.

Open daily from 9:30 A.M. to dusk, with closing hours dependent upon the season. Admission is $8 for adults, $7.25 for seniors, $5.50 for students 6 to 17, $3.25 for children 3 to 5.

## Parks

**Seattle Parks Department,** 100 Dexter Avenue N, Seattle 98109; 206-684-4075.

**Bellevue Parks Department,** P.O. Box 90012, Bellevue 98009; 425-452-2752.

**Discovery Park Visitors' Headquarters,** 3801 W Government Way, Seattle 98199-1014; 206-386-4236.
Open daily from 8:30 A.M. to 5 P.M.

**Kirkland Parks Department,** 425-828-1217.

**Klondike Gold Rush National Historic Park,** 117 S Main Street, Seattle 98104; 206-553-7220.
The museum/park is open from 9 A.M. to 5 P.M. daily except for Thanksgiving, Christmas, and New Year's Day. Admission is free.

**Mercer Slough Nature Trail,** 2102 Bellevue Way SE, Bellevue 98004; 425-452-2752.
The nature trails are open daily, from dawn to dusk. Free guided nature walks are offered Sundays at 11 A.M. Registration is not required. Guided canoe trips on Mercer Slough take place Saturdays from 9 A.M. to noon, from May through

September. Pre-registration is required. Information about canoe and kayak rentals is available by calling 425-637-8838.

**Washington Park Arboretum Visitor Center,** 2300 Arboretum Drive E, Seattle 98112; 266-543-8800. Open weekdays from 10 A.M. to 4 P.M., weekends and holidays from noon to 4 P.M. Admission to the Japanese Garden is $2.50 for adults, $1.50 for students and seniors. Children under 6 admitted free.

## Schools

**Seattle Pacific University,** Third Avenue W and W Nickerson Street, Seattle 98119; 206-281-2000.

**Seattle University,** Broadway and Madison Avenue, Seattle 98122; 206-296-2000.

**University of Washington,** 4014 University Way NE, Seattle 98195; 206-453-2100.

## Shopping

**Alderwood Mall,** 3000 184th Street SW, Lynnwood 98037; 425-771-1211.

**Bellevue Square,** NE Eighth Street and Bellevue Way, Bellevue 98004; 425-454-8096.

**Bon Marche,** 1601 Third Avenue, Seattle 98101; 206-506-6000.

**City Centre,** 1420 Fifth Avenue, Seattle 98101; 206-624-8800.

**Eddie Bauer,** 1330 Fifth Avenue, Seattle 98101; 206-622-2766.

**Gilman Village,** 317 NW Gilman Boulevard, Issaquah 98027; 425-392-6802.

**NIKETOWN,** 1500 Sixth Avenue, Seattle 98101; 206-447-6453.

**Nordstrom,** 1501 Fifth Avenue, Seattle 98101; 206-628-2111.

**Northgate Mall,** 555 Northgate Mall, Seattle 98125; 206-362-4777.

**Pacific Place,** 600 Pine Street, Seattle 98101; 206-405-2655.

**Pike Place Market,** First Avenue and Pike Street, Seattle 98101; 206-682-7453.

**Rainier Square,** 500 Union Street, Seattle 98101; 206-623-0340.

**Recreational Equipment Inc.,** 222 Yale Avenue N, Seattle 98109-5429; 206-223-1944.

**SeaTac Mall,** 1928 S SeaTac Mall, Federal Way 98003; 253-839-6151.

**Southcenter Mall,** 633 Southcenter, Seattle 98188; 206-246-7400.

**SuperMall of the Great Northwest,** 1101 SuperMall Way, Auburn 98001; 253-833-9500.

**University Village,** 2673 NE University Village, Seattle 98105; 206-523-0622.

**Uwajimaya,** 519 Sixth Avenue S, Seattle 98104; 206-624-6248.

**Westlake Center,** 400 Pine Street, Seattle 98101; 206-467-1600.

## Transportation

**Metro Transit,** 206-553-3000.

**Community Transit,** 800-562-1375; 425-778-2185.

**Farwest Taxi,** 206-622-1717.

**Graytop Cab,** 206-282-8222.

**Yellow Cab,** 206-622-6500.

**Shuttle Express,** 805 Lenora Street, Seattle 98121; 206-622-1424.
Provides door-to-door transportation to Sea-Tac International Airport.

**Gray Line of Seattle,** 4500 Marginal Way SW, Seattle 98106; 206-626-5208.

**Victoria Clippers,** 2701 Alaskan Way, Pier 60, Seattle 98121; 206-449-5000.
Provides water transportation to Vancouver Island and Victoria, BC.

**Washington State Ferries,** 801 Alaskan Way, Pier 52/Colman Dock, Seattle 98104; 800-84-FERRY (within Washington) or 206-464-6400.

**Kenmore Air,** 6321 NE 175th Street, Seattle 98155; 425-486-1257.
Offers Seaplane transportation from Seattle to Victoria and the San Juan Islands.

**Amtrak,** 3035 S. Jackson Street, Seattle 98104; 800-872-7245.

## Appendix C: Great Tastes

Listed here are restaurants and cafés, conveniently located along the walk routes, that we particularly recommend if you want to stop for a snack, a full meal, or a dessert-and-coffee break.

### Walk 1

**Desert Fire,** Pacific Place, 600 Pine Street; 206-405-3400.

If you wish to browse the shops of Pacific Place, the hostess at this popular fourth-floor restaurant will equip you with a buzzer that you can put in a pocket or purse. It will sound when your table is ready. Grilled tacos and quesadillas are among the Southwest dishes on the luncheon menu.

**Westlake Center,** 400 Pine Street; 206-467-1600.

The food hall on the Monorail level of the mall features 25 restaurants and food booths.

### Walk 2

**Cutters Market Place Bistro,** 2001 Western Avenue; 206-448-4884.

Northwest seafood is featured in a treasured location, on the fringe of Pike Place Market, overlooking Elliott Bay.

**Copacabana Café,** Pike Place Market; 206-622-6359.

Try a bowl of spicy shrimp soup on a second-story deck that looks out on the Pike Place Market scene.

### Walk 3

**Merchants' Café,** 109 Yesler Way; 206-624-1515.

Try a bowl of salmon chowder or a sandwich at this Pioneer

Square establishment, which opened as the Merchants' Exchange Saloon in 1890.

**Il Terrazzo Carmine,** 411 First Avenue S; 206-467-7797. Some critics rate this the best Italian restaurant in Seattle, and it thrives despite being somewhat hard to find.

## Walk 4

**Queen Anne Café,** 2121 Queen Anne Avenue N; 206-285-2060.
Terrific breakfasts and lunches priced from $5.50 to $8, with the Eggs Benedict particularly recommended. Your coffee cup will never be empty.

**Racha Noodles,** 537 First Avenue N; 206-281-8883.
A place for serious carbohydrate loading. The selection of Thai noodle dishes in the $7 range is varied, filling, and delicious.

## Walk 5

**Still Life in Fremont Coffee House,** 709 N 35th Street; 206-547-9850.
The gathering place of the locals, featuring hearty soups, sandwiches, and homemade desserts served on tables and chairs seemingly rescued from Fremont yard sales.

**The Longshoreman's Daughter Café,** 3508 Fremont Place N; 206-633-5169.
The music is funky, and so are the service and the décor in this oasis for counterculture Fremont residents. But the food—for example, the sweet-potato corn chowder and the shrimp-filled corn cakes with roasted pepper sauce—is pretty good.

## Walk 6

**Chinook's at Salmon Bay,** Fishermen's Terminal, 1900 W
Nickerson Street; 206-283-HOOK.
Some 600 customers a day choose from 100 menu items at
this bustling seafood establishment with a terrific view of
Seattle's commercial fishing fleet. The breakfasts are also
highly recommended.

## Walk 7

**The Point Grill,** 2770 Alki Avenue SW; 206-933-0118.
Indoor and outdoor tables are available on a busy and interesting beach drive. Try the Turkey Mediterranean or grilled
salmon sandwich.

**Spud Fish and Chips,** 2666 Alki Avenue SW; 206-938-
0606.
Possibly the best fish and chips in Seattle. On sunny days,
order to go and picnic across the street, on the beach, or at
one of the tables near the Alki Bath House Art Studio.

## Walk 8

**Byzantion,** 601 Broadway E; 206-325-7580.
The view from sidewalk tables on busy and bizarre Broadway
Avenue is almost as enticing as the menu, which features seven
Greek salads and complete dinners for under $8.

**Chutney's,** 605 15th Avenue E; 206-726-1000.
One of three locations in Seattle where highly acclaimed
Indian cuisine is served under the Chutney's banner. The
food servers will gladly help you select the dish and degree
of heat that suits your tastes.

## Walk 9

**Cactus,** 4220 E Madison Street; 206-324-4140.
Arguably the best Mexican restaurant in Seattle, with specialties ranging from the obligatory tacos and enchiladas to ancho-cinnamon chicken with Navajo fry bread and tortilla-crusted lamb chops.

## Walk 11

**Red Mill Burgers,** 312 N 67th Street; 206-284-6363.
Fast food inside the zoo is uninspired, and the service is often slow. A better choice is to buy a sack of "Verde Burgers with Secret Mill Sauce" at this nearby takeout spot and feast on them at a picnic table inside the zoo. The fries and milkshakes are also first-rate.

## Walk 12

**Six Degrees,** 7900 E Green Lake Drive N; 206-523-1600.
Located just across the street from the Green Lake walking path, this café/pub offers an innovative assortment of salads, sandwiches, and appetizers. For a full meal, try the spicy baked chicken with mashed potatoes.

## Walk 14

**Tokyo Garden,** 4337 University Way NE; 206-632-2014.
From one vantage point on the thoroughfare popularly known as "The Ave," you can spot the signs of seven oriental restaurants, including this one, which serves outstanding teriyaki at bargain prices.

**Pagliacci,** 4529 University Way NE; 206-632-0421.
University students eat a lot of pizza, and this parlor—part
of a local chain—is one of their favorites.


## Walk 16

**Pancake Corral,** 1606 Bellevue Way SE, Bellevue; 425-
454-8888.
Turn right as you leave the Mercer Slough parking lot to
reach this nearby breakfast spot. There are several varieties
of hotcakes plus a daily luncheon special.


## Walk 17

**Kirkland Roaster and Ale House,** 111 Central Way,
Kirkland; 425-325-8486.
Located next to the starting and finishing point of Walk 17,
this restaurant/pub features chicken, beef, and ham cooked
on a 9-foot-high vertical spit roaster.

**Yarrow Bay Grill and Beach Café,** 1270 Carillon Point,
Kirkland; 425-889-9052.
There is formal dining with outstanding seafood upstairs, a
lively crowd and informal atmosphere downstairs. From both
levels, you can enjoy a great view of Lake Washington and
the Carillon Point Marina.


## Walk 18

**Madrona Waterfront Café,** foot of Madison Avenue,
Winslow-Bainbridge Island; 206-842-8339.
It is hard to beat the view from the dining deck above the
Winslow Marina. The crispy fish and chips are above aver-
age, or you can order a complete seafood luncheon entree
for about $8.

## Walk 19

**Forecasters Public House,** 14300 NE 145th Street,
   Woodinville; 425-483-3232.

The public house is part of Redhook Brewery, one of the
walk highlights. You can eat inside or at one of several picnic tables on the banks of the Sammamish River.

**Chateau Ste. Michelle,** 14111 NE 145th Street,
   Woodinville; 425-488-3300.

You can buy picnic items and wine in the winery gift shop
and enjoy it at one of the tables next to the garden or pond.

# Appendix D: Useful Phone Numbers

**Auto Impound:** 206-684-5444

**AAA of Washington:** 206-448-5353

**Better Business Bureau:** 206-448-8888

**Crisis Clinic:** 206-461-3222

**King County Library:** 800-462-9600

**King County Sheriff:** emergency 911, non-emergency 206-296 3311

**Medical Communications Center:** 206-726-2600

**Seattle Police:** emergency 911, non-emergency 206-625 5011

**Weather:** 206-526-6087

**Washington Poison Center:** 206-526-2121

# Appendix E: Read All About It

Want to read more about Seattle and western Washington? The following books are a sample of many you might enjoy.

## Nonfiction

Morgan, Murray C. *Skid Road*. Seattle: University of Washington Press, 1951.

The impact of the lumbering and railroad industries, the Klondike gold rush, and the Great Fire of 1889 are explored in this entertaining history of early Seattle.

Morgan, Murray and Shorett, Alice. *The Pike Place Market, People, Politics and Produce*. Seattle: Pacific Search Press, 1982.

The inside story of one of the world's great marketplaces.

Speidel, William C., Jr. *You Can't Eat Mt. Rainier*. Vashon, WA: Nettle Creek Publishing Co., 1955.

——. *Sons of the Profits or There's No Business Like Grow Business*. Vashon, WA: Nettle Creek Publishing Co., 1967.

——. *Doc Maynard, the Man Who Invented Seattle*. Vashon, WA: Nettle Creek Publishing Co., 1978.

Speidel's irreverent views of Seattle's pioneer period make fascinating reading. His interest in the Pioneer Square area prompted him to create the Underground Tours, which attract thousands of visitors each year.

Steinbrueck, Victor. *Seattle Cityscape*. Seattle: University of Washington Press, 1962.

The architecture and ambiance of Steinbrueck's favorite city are covered in this work by the late professor of urban planning.

Watson, Emmett. *My Life in Print*. Seattle: Lesser Seattle Publishing, 1993.

This longtime Seattle newspaper columnist profiles key figures in Seattle commerce, sports, and politics.

## Fiction

Thesman, Jean. *The Moonstones*. New York: Viking, 1998.

A teenaged heroine finds romance and mystery in an old house on Puget Sound.

Wilbee, Brenda. *Sweetbriar*. Eugene, OR: Harvest House, 1983.

This and two subsequent Sweetbriar novels concern the romance of two actual Seattle pioneers, Louisa Boren and David Denny.

Detective novels by J. A. Jance, Jayne Krentz, Earl Emerson, Stephen Greenleaf, and K.K. Beck have been set in Seattle.

# Appendix F: Local Walking Clubs

The following clubs are all members of the American Volkssport Association, a network of clubs  that sponsor noncompetitive walking, swimming, and bicycling events. To receive information on the AVA or on local clubs call 800-830-WALK or visit the AVA website at www.ava.org.

Most shopping malls in the Seattle area also sponsor walking clubs. See Appendix B for a listing of the larger malls.

**Bellevue Eastside Y,** 10829 NE 19th Place, Bellevue 98004.

**Cascade Ramblers,** 35806 First Avenue S, Federal Way 98003.

**Cedar River Rovers,** 30323 SE 273rd Place, Ravensdale 98051.

**Emerald City Wanderers,** P.O. Box 16221, Seattle 98116.

**Evergreen State Volkssport Association,** 2616 NE 20th Street, Renton 98056.

**Evergreen Wanderers,** P.O. Box 11943, Tacoma 98411.

**Four-Plus Foolhardy Folks,** P.O. Box 424, Renton 98057.

**FS Family Wanderers,** 1627 Fourth Avenue W, Seattle 98119.

**Global Adventurers,** 2023 Aberdeen Avenue SE, Renton 98055-4537.

**Hopkins Telephone Pioneers,** 19905 SE 300th Street, Kent 98042.

**Interlaken Trailblazers,** P.O. Box 40281, Bellevue 98015-4281.

**Mercer Island Volkssport Club,** P.O. Box 1435, Mercer Island 98040-1435.

**Northwest Striders,** 2347 128th Avenue SE, Bellevue 98005-4233.

**Over the Hill Gang,** P.O. Box 23057, Federal Way 98093-0057.

**Puget Sound Sloshers,** P.O. Box 31, Lynnwood 98046-0031.

**Sea-Tac Volkssport Club,** P.O. Box 25101, Federal Way 98093-2101.

**Third Planet Volkstours,** 35806 First Avenue S, Federal Way 98003.

# Index

Page numbers in *italics* refer to photos
Page numbers in **bold** refer to maps

**239**

**241**

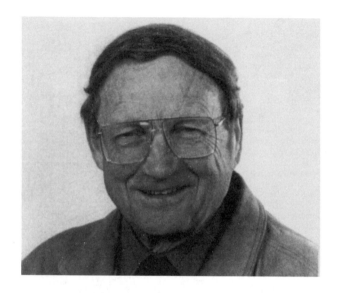

## Meet the Author

A longtime Seattle newspaper columnist, John Owen was named Sportswriter of the Year for the state of Washington on seven occasions. He has written eight books and numerous magazine articles covering the subjects of sports, travel, and food.

As a sportswriter, Owen has covered seven Olympic Games, the Super Bowl, the World Series, the Rose Bowl, the Masters Golf Tournament, the NCAA Final Four, and the U.S. Open tennis finals. He traveled to Zaire in 1974 for the heavyweight championship fight between Muhammad Ali and George Foreman.

The author and his wife Alice, a professional artist, are enthusiastic hikers, bicyclists, and cross-country skiers. They have walked the thoroughfares and back streets of 20 foreign countries.

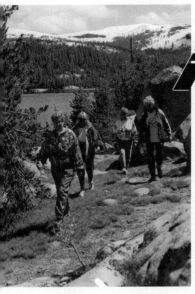

**A WHOLE DIFFERENT KIND OF WALK**

# Experience A Whole Different Kind of Walk

*The American Volkssport Association, America's premier walking organization, provides noncompetitive sporting events for outdoor enthusiasts. More than 500 volkssport (translated "sport of the people") clubs sponsor walks in scenic and historic areas nationwide. Earn special awards for your participation.*

**For a free general information packet, including a listing of clubs in your state, call 1-800-830-WALK (1-800-830-9255).**

*American Volkssport Association is a nonprofit, tax-exempt, national organization dedicated to promoting the benefits of health and physical fitness for people of all ages.*